THE
CLINICAL RESEARCH
SURVIVAL GUIDE

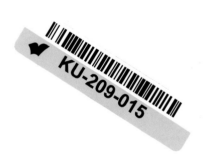

Published by the REMEDICA Group
REMEDICA Publishing Ltd, 32–38 Osnaburgh Street,
London, NW1 3ND, UK

REMEDICA Inc, Tri-State International Center,
Building 25, Suite 150, Lincolnshire,
IL 60069, USA

TC00493

E-mail: books@remedica.com
www.remedica.com

Publisher: Andrew Ward
In-house editors: Roisin O'Brien, Tamsin White, and Tonya Berthoud
Design: REGRAPHICA, London, UK

ISBN 1 901346 44 7
British Library Cataloguing-in Publication Data
A catalogue record for this book is available from the British Library

Printed & Bound in India by Ajanta Offset.

THE CLINICAL RESEARCH SURVIVAL GUIDE

EDITOR
JOSEF NIEBAUER MD, PHD

University of Leipzig – Heart Center
Germany

Contributors

Editor

Josef Niebauer, MD, PhD
Privatdozent and Consultant Cardiologist
Department of Internal Medicine and Cardiology
University of Leipzig – Heart Center
Strümpellstr. 39
04289 Leipzig
Germany

Authors

Philippa Easterbrook, FRCP, MPH, DTM&H
Professor of HIV/GU Medicine
Weston Education Centre
King's College Hospital
Cutcombe Road
London SE5 9RS
UK

David Lalloo, MBBS, MD, FRCP
Senior Lecturer and Honorary Consultant Physician
Liverpool School of Tropical Medicine
Pembroke Place
Liverpool L3 5QA
UK

Andrew J Maxwell, MD, FACC
Stanford University
Division of Pediatric Cardiology
750 Welch Road, Suite 305
Palo Alto, CA 94304
USA

Paul G McNally, MD, FRCP
Department of Diabetes and Endocrinology
Leicester Royal Infirmary
University Hospitals of Leicester NHS Trust
Leicester
LE1 5WW
UK

Graeme Moyle, MBBS, MD
Associate Director of HIV Research
Chelsea and Westminster Hospital
369 Fulham Road
London
SW10 9NH, UK

David L Rowland, PhD
Professor of Psychology
Dean of Graduate Studies
Kretzmann Hall, 116
Valparaiso University
Valparaiso
IN 46383
USA

James A Thornton, PhD
Professor and Director of Graduate Programs in Economics
Eastern Michigan University
Ypsilanti
MI 48197
USA

Charles Weijer, MD, PhD
Associate Professor of Medicine
Department of Bioethics
Halifax, Nova Scotia
Canada
B3H 4H7

Contents

CHAPTER 1
Introduction

Josef Niebauer

Clinical research is essential for medical progress and the subsequent delivery of the best possible care to patients. With the advent of evidence-based medicine (EBM), the search for the right clinical foundation upon which to base therapeutic interventions is intensifying. The drive for objectivity and sound guidelines is being fuelled by solid data acquired in correctly performed clinical trials. This leaves less scope for clinicians to base treatments solely on personal experience or recommendations from colleagues. Certainly, experience will remain invaluable, perhaps even inspirational, but knowledge so generated will inevitably be limited in comparison with that gained from several hundred investigators taking part in multi-center trials. Not only do such studies provide a direct link to greater knowledge, they also make it possible to compare individual experiences with trial findings and re-assess treatment options—a boon in helping to prevent personal views and strategies from becoming too restrictive.

It has been said "to a man with a hammer, everything looks like a nail". As a result of clinical trials, we can not only analyze our own decision making, but also consider the advice of experts we could otherwise never consult.

Although clinicians should use EBM as the bedrock of decision making, application of ethical values, judgment and face-to-face assessment of the patient are equally important. A good knowledge of the essentials of clinical research should help to prevent over-interpretation of results by clinicians.

Career opportunities in medicine are becoming very limited and there is an increasing necessity to obtain additional qualifications and bolster one's curriculum vitae with research experience and publications. Successful performance in clinical research and clinical trials has opened doors for many physicians in the past and will continue to do so in the future. This is true for all the authors of this book. One of the purposes of this book is to point colleagues in the right direction and to help them make the most of their research experience. This book will benefit those who:

- have never done any clinical research but would like to

- have done some clinical research and want to take it further

- see their future success primarily in terms of clinical research

By emphasizing the importance of clinical research, the authors hope to help colleagues enjoy, as well as succeed in, research. It will be a bonus if readers gain a greater understanding of those scientists and clinicians who are trying to push further forward the frontiers of knowledge.

CHAPTER 2
Why clinical research?
David Lalloo

People are motivated to do research for many different reasons. Some are driven by pure curiosity and a genuine desire to spend most of their working life advancing medical knowledge. Others seek fame and fortune, although these are extremely difficult to find. However, for most of us, research is just one aspect of a predominantly clinical career—albeit one that all of us need to consider at certain times. Why do it?

For many, the initial stimulus for considering research is the desire to further their careers. There can be no doubt that possession of a research degree and/or publications will make you more employable and may be a prerequisite for a decent job in some highly competitive specialties. There has been much criticism of the amount of poor quality research that this need to 'bolster' the curriculum vitae has produced. Certainly, entering research without a real desire to do well and without interest in your research project may lead to a number of unhappy years and is unlikely to be productive. This should be avoided at all costs. On the other hand, many medical graduates who have been introduced to research by the need to advance their careers have enjoyed it immensely and some have been stimulated to take up an academic career as a result. The crucial thing is to find a project that you are interested in and to be quite clear what you want to gain from your period of research.

Basic or clinical science?
One of the first decisions to make is choosing between basic scientific or clinical research. The advent of new molecular techniques has considerably expanded the scope and

opportunities for basic scientific research. As a result, people interested in basic research now have a genuine choice about the type of research that they can do. Realistically, a lot depends upon the opportunities that exist at the time that you decide to become involved in research. However, there are some essential considerations. Basic scientific research will be a completely new venture. You will be taken from an environment in which you are reasonably competent to a laboratory in which everything is foreign and unfamiliar. Inevitably, this means that it will take you some time to learn techniques and adjust to a new working pattern. Some people find this adaptation difficult and have problems seeing the relevance of the work that they are doing to their major interest in clinical medicine. However, for others, the pure focus on asking questions and solving them in the laboratory is far more intellectually stimulating and, therefore, motivating because it is so different from their normal clinical work. Freedom from the stresses and strains of face-to-face contact with patients may be just what is needed to recharge the intellectual batteries. You need to decide which of these situations are likely to apply to you. One thing is certain, it is extremely difficult, without prior training, to consider engaging in basic research for short periods of time. Successful science can hardly ever be performed when there are significant clinical commitments. Most people spend 2–3 years in a laboratory and you need to be committed to your project to make it work.

Clinical research is slightly different. Research projects can be completed in a shorter period of time, as some of the skills will be familiar to you and far less time needs to be spent learning the ropes. Many find clinical research more motivating than laboratory research; it is generally easier to see how the results of your efforts will directly affect, and hopefully improve, patient care. However, in the era of molecular medicine, clinical research is not an easy option. It is probably harder to find a good clinical research project than it is to find a good laboratory-based project. Really successful clinical research often incorporates a great deal of collaboration with other investigators—it may be more difficult to have a clearly defined project that is your own. The very nature of dealing with clinical subjects adds additional problems to the difficulties of research; in the laboratory you rarely need to worry about ethics committees; the difficulty of informed consent and recruitment of patients; patients returning for follow-up; and other similar considerations. However, clinical research does allow you to build upon the skills that you have already acquired, develop new skills that are more easily applicable to the clinical world and may better prepare you for a subsequent clinical career.

What do you gain from clinical research?

Even though clinical research still involves patient contact, many clinicians find a period of time spent away from the hurly-burly of continuous service commitments refreshing. As an individual progresses through medical school and postgraduate education, much of their training is dependent upon the learning of facts, often without a great deal of intellectual input. A period in clinical research allows you to think about clinical medicine and practice in a very different way. The discipline of defining clinical questions and thinking how you might answer those questions, allows you to approach clinical problems in a far more analytical fashion. Ultimately, you will develop skills in critical thinking that are not part of standard training and these often change peoples' approach to clinical practice. You also have time to think about one area of your specialty in depth rather than the superficial knowledge of many subjects that is necessary to practice everyday medicine. For many, it is a chance to build up a body of knowledge and develop an area of special expertise which continues for the rest of your clinical career.

The other advantage of clinical research is learning about clinical trials. There is no doubt that the best way to learn about clinical trials is to be involved in them. The mysteries of case-control and cohort studies become much clearer once you are forced to think about the design of a study that you are interested in.

Similarly, comprehension of data analysis and medical statistics often only become really clear when you start to analyze your own data and become involved practically in selecting the appropriate methods to do so.

---

focus on...
EVIDENCE-BASED MEDICINE

WHAT IS IT?

Evidence-based medicine (EBM) has been defined as: "the conscientious, explicit and judicious use of current best evidence in making decisions about the care of individual patients". That is, 'good' doctors should integrate individual clinical expertise with the best available external clinical evidence. This integration is essential. After all, evidence is fine when applied appropriately, but there are likely to be patients for whom it is not appropriate—consider the inclusion and exclusion criteria of many of the major trials. However, without a knowledge of current best evidence, your patients may suffer as your clinical practice becomes dated. Although it should be possible to argue that everyone should already be practicing such an approach, alas this is certainly not the case. When you consider simply the number of clinical trials published in any year in any one therapeutic area, it is not surprising that keeping abreast of the 'best available external clinical evidence' is a difficult task. Since 'best available external clinical evidence' is certainly not restricted to reports of properly conducted clinical trials, the task becomes even more difficult. Even so, there are instances of successfully applied EBM and doctors should strive to practice it.

Are there any advantages in knowing about clinical trials? Even if research has never really appealed to you, there is no doubt that clinical decision making is becoming increasingly based on good clinical trial evidence. It is likely that the techniques of evidence-based medicine (EBM) will become prerequisites for good clinical practice over the next couple of decades. While EBM can certainly be learnt without performing clinical trials, involvement in clinical research can only help in this regard. Time spent in clinical research will help you to read and analyze the medical literature more coherently, learn the computer skills that are increasingly necessary in the practice of medicine today and become more focused and logical in the way that you approach difficult and challenging clinical problems.

Fitting clinical research into your career

How does clinical research fit into career plans? For the die-hard basic or clinical scientist for whom the thrill and satisfaction of generating hypotheses, designing experiments to test those hypotheses and publishing the results are the major motivating factors, two main paths are available.

The first path is the standard academic route dependent upon the acquisition of long-term grants to fund clinical research and sometimes your salary. It must be said that in today's increasingly competitive environment, only those at the absolute top of their field can see this as a permanent career path. It is also fair to say that this is unlikely to make you rich. The second path is to join the commercial sector, usually a pharmaceutical company. This environment is likely to be more financially rewarding, but a company's research priorities are unlikely to be the same as your own and the level of job security is unlikely to be high.

The potential personal rewards from participation in successful clinical research should not be under-estimated. A great deal of satisfaction can be gained from the development of skills that allow the formulation of research questions and the design of trials to answer those questions. For many, clinical research activity is one of the most rewarding aspects of their professional practice.

Clearly, if you intend to become an academic, much of your training will be research-based and some doctors now choose either a combined MD/PhD course or do a PhD in between their pre-clinical and clinical training. However, remember that unless you really want to be a pure scientist, clinical training and experience will help you to identify important clinical problems to study and provide you with an alternative career structure, should research impetus become difficult to maintain. Research also requires people who can sit happily at the interface between clinical medicine and pure science; clinical training prepares you perfectly to fulfill this role. It is extremely difficult to be a good clinical research academic without spending a substantial amount of time in clinical training. Therefore, most of us will want to integrate research training with clinical training. What is the best way to do this?

The UK experience

The advent of the Calman training scheme has clearly changed things for most specialties as the traditional Research Registrar position between Registrar and Senior Registrar posts is no longer appropriate. The Calman scheme is a higher specialty training program which usually lasts 4–5 years. To enter the scheme, trainees compete at interview for a Specialist Registrar post and national training number (NTN), which ultimately lead to a specialist qualification, the Certificate of Completion of Specialist Training (CCST).

As a trainee, there are now two points during the course of your career when you might consider research. The first is after the completion of general professional training, i.e. before starting a Calman training scheme. If a reasonable amount of time (2–3 years) is spent in research at this point, it has the advantage of putting you in a strong position to apply for a Specialist Registrar post on a Calman scheme, especially in the competitive specialties. However, it also means that your exposure to the specialty of your choice has probably been limited. It is unlikely that you will have had a chance to develop an interest in aspects of your specialty that will have led to the generation of research ideas or projects that you may want to follow through.

Most doctors will undertake research during the period of Calman training. Although the scheme is still in its early stages and it is too early to say how the integration of research into Calman will truly work, there are two theoretical ways of carrying out research as part of a Specialist Registrar training scheme. Most training schemes allow at least a year of research to count towards training for a CCST. If your aim is to learn a little about research methodology and gain some of the benefits of clinical research training that have been outlined above, then this may be possible within existing schemes with the permission of the Postgraduate Dean and your specialty advisor. A short period such as a year is unlikely to allow you much time to perform work in the laboratory and is, therefore, best suited to fitting in with existing clinical research projects in the department.

If your aim is to complete the 2–3 years necessary to obtain an MD or PhD, then you are likely to need external funding from either funding agencies or drug companies. These longer research periods are permitted within Calman and you can keep a training number during such periods with the agreement of the Postgraduate Dean. However, it is most unlikely that departments will pay a salary during this time. This in theory should allow you more freedom to pursue research projects that are of particular interest to you, but, in practice, most Research Registrars end up with projects that reflect the research areas and interests of the group that they are working with. The opportunities open to a trainee depend upon both different specialties and the departments within that specialty. Therefore, it is crucial that you make enquiries about research opportunities and areas of research interest when you consider a Specialist Registrar post in a particular unit.

It is essential that you consider a clinical research post carefully. Although you will gain some of the benefits of research from any post, some positions will be much more beneficial, both personally and professionally, than others. The importance of being interested in the proposed project cannot be over-emphasized. It may be tempting to accept the project that is handed to you on a plate by your boss, but unless the subject really stimulates you, things are unlikely to go well. Does your proposed supervisor have a good record for gaining grants and producing publications? Does he/she look after his/her Research Registrars? Will you actually be trained to use specific research techniques or will you be left to your own devices? Opportunities to go on statistics or epidemiology courses, or to travel to conferences are extremely helpful. Many of these questions are best answered by existing or previous Research Registrars in the same unit.

Much of the best clinical research is collaborative across a number of centers. You need to be sure that there is a clearly defined role for you in a project, which will lead to a body of work that you can write up as a thesis. If work is to be shared with others, for which sections will you be responsible and will you be a first author on some of the papers that emerge?

focus on...
MONEY

In the real world, although the greatest incentive to physicians taking part in a sponsored trial is probably the money, many are genuinely interested in the question being addressed. Clinical trial duties need to be conducted on top of what is already likely to be a very busy schedule and so are unlikely to be undertaken without a sufficiently attractive financial reward as well as the personal satisfaction gained from the research. Such monies can then be channeled into the investigator's own research projects, into a travel fund or be used to buy new equipment. Not all physicians are driven exclusively by the financial arrangements but where money is involved, unfortunately, there is the potential for abuse. Payments on a per patient basis could lead to the enrolment of unsuitable subjects (e.g. those not meeting the exclusion or inclusion criteria) and the pharmaceutical sponsor making large payments for little or no return. A more satisfactory arrangement is for the pharmaceutical sponsor to pay only for evaluable patients, i.e. those who satisfy the exclusion and inclusion criteria and are randomized into the trial. Payments are generally determined on a trial-by-trial basis and are likely to vary between sponsors and therapeutic areas. However, money may not be all that physicians obtain from a sponsor. Some companies offer various ancillary services as an adjunct or supplement to the money. Staff training is a valuable service, facilitating both the current trial and possible future trials. The sponsor may also pay for new equipment or for the provision of a research nurse for the duration of the study. Such 'extras' are very valuable and should be considered alongside any financial offer from the company.

WHERE DOES THE MONEY GO?
You also need to be aware that, in an increasingly commercial environment, your hospital is likely to want to see a share of the proceeds from your participation in a trial. Some levy a flat-rate fee for equipment use—it's not 'your' equipment and extra usage in a trial is likely to lead to increased maintenance costs, etc. Similarly, the pharmacy and laboratory may wish to charge for their services. Make sure before you agree to participate in a trial that you find out what you will be charged by the hospital and other departments—then work out whether you can afford to take part.

Successful research is a full-time occupation. You should keep routine clinical commitments to a minimum; an apparently 'light' commitment of two or three out-patient clinics a week will interfere seriously with your ability to perform good research. Checking such facts, and clarifying the expectations of your supervisor before taking up a research post, can prevent many problems and sometimes unpleasantness later.

Be realistic

It is important to recognize that there are disadvantages as well as advantages to spending time in research. You are likely to experience a drop in salary during your research post unless you continue on-call commitments. Most academics are restricted in the amount of private practice that they can do. There are, therefore, financial disadvantages to spending time in research on both a short- and long-term basis. Unfortunately, this lack of financial reward is not because research is an easier option or involves less work. In fact, most find that they work longer hours in research than they ever did in their clinical posts. The distinction between work and home life is far more blurred; there are always papers to be read or data to be analyzed. Although research offers a far more flexible lifestyle, some become stressed by the feeling that there is always something to be done. There is also a constant pressure to produce results, both from your boss and because you are aware of the need to produce publications. Almost everyone goes through phases when they wish that they had stuck to the simpler less stressful life of clinical medicine. However, most doctors ultimately emerge from a period of clinical research feeling that they have gained a great deal personally and professionally. Many feel that they are far better doctors as a consequence of their research training. At the very least, all of us should think seriously about spending some time in clinical research as part of our training.

Further reading

Cox TM. The academic clinician. Journal of the Royal College of Physicians 1999;33:411–3.

Royal College of Physicians. Guidelines for clinicians entering research, 1997.

CHAPTER 3
The US experience
Andrew Maxwell

The reasons for participating in clinical research, as well as how and when to fit research into a career, are universal. However, the details of how to go about beginning and cultivating a career involving research are quite different in the US and the UK.

Beginning a career

Some know that they are destined for a career in research early in their training. For these individuals, participation in a research project during their college years is a very good idea. Exposure to research during this time can help to determine early whether or not they are suited to a research life. This experience can help individuals to determine with confidence whether pursuit of a PhD, with the great commitment involved, is right for them. This is also important for those who have chosen to apply for medical school. If research is likely to be a significant portion of a future career, applying for a combined MD/PhD is a way to achieve both degrees in a relatively short period of time; often the two degrees can be obtained in as little as 5–6 years. This is not to say that early career development should be rushed, but, in the highly competitive world of research, the possession of either a PhD or an MD/PhD can provide the 'clout' necessary for the acquisition of grants and postdoctoral positions which can then be undertaken at a reasonable pace. The other reason to pursue research during college years is that the experience and any publications gained may help to secure a highly coveted spot in a prestigious predoctoral training program.

For those wishing to become involved in research during their college years, the selection of a project is not nearly as important as the selection of a mentor. Indeed, selection of a project in a field outside of where an ultimate interest may lie can provide the opportunity to bring unique tools and perspectives into a preferred field in the next stage of an individual's career. Mentor selection during college years is mainly an issue of compatibility. A healthy relationship between the student and mentor is extremely important. As well as offering the opportunity for the casual dissemination of information about how to succeed in research, a healthy relationship should result in a good letter of recommendation and even a proactive participation by the mentor in securing a spot in a training program. Of course, the chance of receiving these benefits is also directly related to the time that is put into the project; it is often late at night or over the weekend when the mentor takes an interest in imparting knowledge helpful to the student, and it is these hours that are remembered when the mentor gauges the enthusiasm of his/her recommendation. When a mentor is selected, after considering compatibility, his/her track record of mentoring should be scrutinized. Has he/she provided worthwhile projects, i.e. those leading to publications, to former students? Is he/she sufficiently respected and actively contributing in the field such that a recommendation is meaningful to a training program? This may be answered by determining where former students are now. At this early stage of development, the mentor's track record of grant acquisition is only important to the extent that it helps determine his/her standing in the scientific community; it is unlikely that significant financial support for a student to participate in research will be forthcoming at this stage. Having said this, the US National Institutes of Health (NIH) does provide an opportunity for third and fourth year students to compete for the Undergraduate Training Grant (T34) which provides up to 2 years of stipend and tuition assistance for projects. There is also a very good Summer Internship Program in Biomedical Research [1] for college students at the NIH campus in Bethesda, Maryland and other select locations.

For those wishing to become involved in research during their medical school or residency years, the advice given for college years still applies. However, there is an obvious advantage if the choice of mentor is restricted to the field of medicine that the student ultimately chooses to pursue. In this regard, it often makes sense to commence research following the general clinical internship/residency. Taking a year or two to conduct research in a field intended as a sub-specialty may result in a strong recommendation from someone well-known in the field, which may help in securing a spot in a highly desired fellowship. However, this advantage should be considered in the context of the type of relationship that the individual might ultimately have with his/her research group. Is it better to be a tiny unmemorable cog in the research machine of a Nobel prize winner who is always away on the lecture circuit, or to be the key player in the success of an up-and-coming group conducting research that may be outside an immediate field of interest but that may enable familiarization with tools whose use could expand research within an ultimate research field?

During this stage of development, unless time is taken off, support for research participation is rare. The NIH does provide opportunities for medical students to participate in a Summer Research Fellowship Program (SRFP) [2] in Bethesda, Maryland and other select locations. If the medical student elects to take a year or two off, there are additional funding opportunities. Grant support should be expected by the student in this case and should either be provided by pre-arrangement with the mentor through one of his/her grants or through application for a Postbaccalaureate Intramural Research Training Award (IRTA) through the NIH. Those who have completed or elected to take time off from medical school or residency may also apply through the NIH for individual and institutional National Research Service Awards (NRSA or T32). These grants provide up to 5 years of support for research activity as long as it is not part of a formal degree seeking program. The process of obtaining the institutional grants in particular is uncomplicated and usually does not require a lengthy lead-time compared to most grant application processes.

For many in medical training, a research career does not begin until either a research requirement is imposed as part of a fellowship or the individual has determined that their specific field of interest is sufficiently compelling to begin contributing to its advancement. At this point, it is probably accurate to say that the project selected is more important than selection of the mentor: it is often the research that serves to introduce the trainee to the scientific community at large. While it is still important that the budding researcher focuses on learning research methodology and tools, it is publication and presentation of research that begin to define his/her career. To be successful, publications and presentations over time should tell a story of advancement in the field. Participation in national conferences as a presenter or in the audience is essential. This is the way to become recognized as part of the scientific community and eventually a thought leader in that field.

Often, research projects are woven into the clinical fellowship and are supported as part of the general fellowship stipend. However, many fellowship programs have the expectation that the final year is used mainly for research and that outside funding is to be secured by the fellow. Financial support for this period is often obtained from the NIH institutional or individual NRSA training grants. However, awards are also available from specific foundations that fund research for their cause such as the American Heart Association or the Robert Wood Johnson Foundation. In addition, established investigators will often have grants from pharmaceutical companies or Program Project Grants that provide funding for unspecified researchers added to a project.

Advancing in research

If, after a few years of mentored research, the intention is to pursue research further, plans to obtain extended support must begin. Career level grants are available that can be applied for. Preparation for a successful grant application begins to take place during the previous years of research. The techniques previously learned, the collaborations made and the demonstration of successful research through publications go a long way in building the foundation of the grant application. At this stage of development, it would be normal to continue mentored research. Thus, the grants applied for at this stage would require a senior investigator, in many institutions a full professor, to be the principal investigator. Examples include the NIH Mentored Clinical Scientist Development Award (K08), which provides up to 5 years of supervised basic science or clinical research, or the NIH Mentored Patient-Oriented Research Career Development Award (K23) [3], which is specific for clinical research. Specific disease foundations also commonly provide grants at this level. Finally, some investigators successfully compete for stipends awarded for outstanding work completed to support further work in the field.

Becoming an independent, non-mentored investigator is the next stage of the career. This usually occurs around year 5 of mentored research. Within academic institutions there are often time requirements for achievement of associate or full professor status before the application for independent funding is allowed. Notwithstanding institutional restrictions, grants as the principal investigator can be applied for at this point. This is an ideal time to apply for the NIH First Independent Research Support and Transition (FIRST) Award (R29) or directly submit for an NIH Investigator Initiated Research Award (R01). Investigators can also begin to participate in collaborative grants such as the NIH Interactive Research Project Grant (IRPG), which is the coordinated submission of two or more related R01s, FIRSTs or institution-wide Program Project Grants (P01). IRPGs award funding for a broadly based multidisciplinary research program that has a well-defined central research focus or objective. Support also continues to be available from private foundations, with these usually increasing in size and term with the growth of the investigator. Finally, pharmaceutical companies may also approach the academic investigator at this stage with the hope that they will perform studies in exchange for grants.

Outside academia

It is becoming more and more popular for academic investigators to look beyond academic recognition as the motivation for their research. Patenting of new techniques, devices, assays, drugs, drug targets, delivery vehicles and gene sequences (amongst other things) is very big business for academic institutions and private businesses alike. It is also becoming popular for academic researchers to license their technology from institutions and to create start-up companies. This can be very rewarding in many respects including:

- the gratification that comes from taking an idea developed in the laboratory to widespread use for the relief of disease

- the pleasure of wearing the many hats of entrepreneur, businessperson, fundraiser and Wall Street pundit

- the potential for great financial gain

The rewards of this route must be weighed against the potential dangers of such a venture, which include:

- great personal and investor debt generated in the early stages from enormous patent and start-up expenses

- the subjection to academic jealousy and disdain for 'going commercial'

- the very real probability of business failure with the anger of financiers and friends who have lost their investment

The support for such a venture does not need to be carried entirely on the back of the founding investigator nor does his/her soul need to be sold to venture capital. A very prudent way to begin developing a successful company centered around an idea from the lab is to apply for an NIH Small Business Innovative Research (SBIR) grant. These grants can provide nearly 1 million dollars (US) over 3 years for the development of a worthwhile idea. The grant is given in two parts: the first part (up to $100,000) is to produce proof-of-concept data in preparation for the second part (up to $750,000). In return for funding, the company must agree to commit an equal amount of money towards the regulatory and marketing costs of the product.

Whether interested in this route or not, it is a very good idea to become familiar with some basic patent laws. All too often, investigators rush to publish abstracts or orally present their new findings without first stopping by their institution's office of technology licensing only to realize belatedly that they have created 'prior art' of their work, thereby jeopardizing its patent potential. The investigator may also be tempted to keep a potential invention hidden from the institution where he/she is employed in an effort to reap all the rewards. Here I give a strong word of advice; "Give to Caesar what is Caesar's". The office of technology licensing can aid immensely in sharing the risk borne by patent expenses, can help expedite the patent process, and can assist in finding licensees. These advantages alone are worth the cost of shared royalties. Contrast this with the fact that any invention patented outside the institution that produces substantial royalties will probably be investigated by the institution's licensing office, thereby jeopardizing not only the investigator's job but also his/her standing as a citizen.

For many, a career in academic research is often followed by a career in industry research. While there are academic zealots who frown upon this route, it should be noted that industry research has many positive aspects that contribute to the greater good of disease treatment and prevention. The competitive nature of industry-based research means that all necessary time and resources will be expended on projects that appear very worthwhile, whereas little time will be allowed to be wasted on projects that are not. Industry research also has the advantage of offering immediate and sufficient funding of an important project without the need for the very long, and often disappointing, grant application process. Furthermore, many positions in industry allow for substantial academic freedom. Indeed, competition in industry forces companies to work on basic science questions whereas the scientist in an academic institution must accomplish this with all of his/her competing responsibilities. In general, those who developed their careers in basic science research are well suited for industry drug discovery programs while those who have developed careers in clinical research may find that Phase II and III clinical trial development is more suitable to their tastes.

Summary

While the reasons for pursuing a research career may be universal, the methods of going about developing a career are unique to location. Opportunities in the US are plentiful, not only for the support of research training (no matter what career level the individual chooses to become involved), but also for the direction taken for career development. Great reward opportunities exist including spiritual satisfaction, fame, fortune and sometimes a combination of the three.

References

1   http://www.training.nih.gov/student/internship/info.asp

2   http://www.training.nih.gov/student/srfp/index.asp

3   http://grants.nih.gov/training/careerdevelopmentawards.htm

CHAPTER 4
How to get started in clinical research
Paul McNally

After deciding that clinical research is a route you wish to take, how do you get started? This can be extremely difficult for the novice, but the first, and most important step, is to decide what you would like to do, often with the guidance of an experienced researcher, and to start developing a research plan. Time spent setting up and developing a good project will reap benefits in due course. A project may not come to fruition if essential planning is not done, potential difficulties are not anticipated or funding is not obtained. A clear question must therefore be tabled before a clinical research project is undertaken and a plan of research must be developed before starting. Important questions need to be addressed at the outset and going through this process will prove helpful in the long term.

What can you do?

It is unusual for someone entering clinical research for the first time to generate an idea. You may be bright, but expert help will be needed. Joining a research team with a proven track record and line of research often allows the novice researcher to work on an existing project. This approach will allow the rapid acquisition of new skills and the ability to become familiar with the important questions that need to be answered in that particular field of research.

How do you go about joining a research unit? This is often a high hurdle, but there are various routes you can take. Many research opportunities are advertised in medical journals and the competition may be strong. Other positions may be filled by word of mouth. For those interested in undertaking research, a useful tip is to talk to a known researcher, either in your hospital or university, and let them know you are keen. Researchers often write applications for funding, but do not always have a person in mind to carry out the work. You may find that having expressed an interest, your name is part of the application! This approach tends to lead to more prolonged periods of research time, usually in the region of 2–3 years. It should also be remembered that many departments have research funds available to help pump prime projects. Much of this funding is provided via charitable means or pharmaceutical institutions. It does not matter where this funding comes from, it is much more important to get your research going. Remember, many research applications, no matter how good or how well they score, do not get funded. Do not give up at the first hurdle.

For those not in a dedicated research environment, starting out can be difficult and daunting. Nonetheless, remember that clinical research takes many forms and could involve either an audit project of a particular condition and its outcome or an interesting case history. The latter have their merits and by gaining some basic research experience you will be more attractive for positions in dedicated research units. Clinical audit research is important, particularly in the era of evidence-based practice. Dissemination of morbidity and mortality outcomes for a particular procedure or condition is valuable clinical research and allows comparison of new techniques or procedures with old. Furthermore, with the introduction in the UK of clinical

Pre-testing (and Rehearsing) the Protocol

With the use of new testing instruments and procedures, it is critical to learn about potential problems prior to the onset of the study. A small sample of pilot subjects (which may include colleagues and even oneself) typically provides insight into the kinds of problems that are likely to arise during the test protocol. It is possible to save a lot of time and post-experiment anxiety by ensuring that the protocol generates data that are ultimately meaningful and reliable.

governance (provision of a high quality and accountable service), units will need to benchmark their performance against other services. Straightforward clinical case reports may shed light on rare conditions or novel therapeutic possibilities and are often published in high-impact journals. Whatever avenue you decide to take, it is important to remember that clinical research takes many forms and does not necessarily require technical expertise or funding. Basic library skills are a vital technique needed to allow you to search the literature. Life has been made easier in recent years by the development of literature databases, for example Medline and the internet.

Can you do it?

The complexity of the research you wish to undertake will depend on the facilities available within your research unit. It would, for example, be impossible to undertake a clinical therapeutic drug trial without having the appropriate patients to study. A clinical study requiring the use of laboratory techniques will fail without access to local expertise to teach you the techniques or experts willing to collaborate.

focus on...
THE COORDINATING CENTER

WHAT IS IT?

In multi-center trials, one investigator is often assigned the responsibility for the coordination of investigators at different sites. This investigator is known as the coordinating investigator and their site as the coordinating center.

WHAT DOES IT DO?

The coordinating center can serve a whole range of functions, including trial design, coordination, data management, on-site monitoring of data quality and statistical analysis. Centralization facilitates standardization of procedures. In addition, having one's peers chase you up when there are delays or problems may be more acceptable than having this function performed by a clinical research organization or pharmaceutical sponsor.

Furthermore, collecting the clinical material and taking it to a researcher who has not been involved in the planning of the research project may fail simply because the samples have been collected inappropriately. Seeking help at an early stage of a research project may enthuse others to be part of the project and identify potential problems further down the line. Consultation with a local expert or colleague may raise other important questions that are easy to answer without necessarily complicating the research project—this scenario frequently arises and should not be discouraged. You may have started out with one question to answer, but by the end you may have addressed several important issues related to whatever you are studying. Most researchers do it because they enjoy it. However,

---

focus on...
ARCHIVING

WHAT IS IT?
Clinical trials generate a lot of data and documentation. In order to comply with national guidelines, both sponsor and investigator need to file and retain large amounts of this documentation for what can be a considerable length of time—this process is termed 'archiving'.

WHY IS IT NECESSARY?
Trial documentation may need to be revisited for a number of reasons:

- to satisfy regulatory authorities that the study was carried out according to the guidelines in force during the lifetime of the trial. In the event of an audit, all documentation should be available to allow an inspector to trace a clinical trial from inception to final report, thereby assuring that the study was conducted to the standards demanded

- for re-analysis; from time to time new questions may arise that can only be answered by referring back to original documents

- to ensure that a full description of the study is available in case the study needs to be repeated or to facilitate further work

- to support license applications in other regions and possibly also other indications or therapeutic areas

WHAT NEEDS TO BE ARCHIVED?
All trial documentation needs to be kept until you are informed otherwise by the trial sponsor.

HOW LONG DO I NEED TO KEEP DOCUMENTS FOR?
The trial sponsor is legally obliged to retain all trial documents until 2 years after the last marketing authorization in the International Conference on Harmonization (ICH) region.

As investigator, according to EC guidelines, you need to store clinical trial data for at least 15 years (yes, fifteen). Requirements may vary from country to country, so check with the clinical trials monitor. Archiving also requires appropriate storage facilities and appropriate space, so before the trial you must ensure that you have the capacity to archive (filing cabinets) and a secure room in which to store the archived materials. Plus, you will need this space for 15 years....

at the end of the day, everyone is hoping for at least one publication in a peer-reviewed journal. Consider undertaking a pilot study before venturing into the main study; this will clarify difficult areas with regard to data collection. In a clinical research audit, for instance, documenting information from clinical records may sound easy, but if the data are not documented routinely, the audit project will fail. This is particularly true for medical records as note-taking and documentation of results are often badly performed, not done at all or missing. Equally, a laboratory-based study might involve developing or fine-tuning a biochemical assay. Thus, a pilot run may identify at an early stage that the planned project is not viable, saving time in the long term and hopefully maintaining your enthusiasm.

Clinical studies involving patients warrant special attention. Recruiting patients is the hardest part of any study. Well-informed patients are more likely to participate. Patient information leaflets and posters in clinic areas are helpful. Recruitment tends to be more successful if conducted on a personal level, rather than by letter alone. For pharmaceutical therapeutic trials, patient information leaflets may need to be modified for local use or translated into other languages. Remember to inform colleagues to look for suitable patients. Consider preparing a one-sided A4 summary of the study and recruitment criteria for the clinic to remind everyone to be on the look out for subjects. Electronic searching of patient clinical information systems or manual searching of medical records before the patient comes for a routine visit may help identification and bring patients to the attention of the investigator, for example by attaching a sticker to the front of their notes. Remember that patients often have frequent visits to hospital specialists, professions allied to medicine, as well as to primary care. Therefore, be flexible in scheduling patients, otherwise recruitment will be unsuccessful or they will drop out. Combining routine clinics with the study will save the patient unnecessary visits. Stress the benefits of enrollment into a study stating, for example, that they might receive a very detailed assessment of their medical condition. Always start the first few visits of a study with one or two patients at the most so that you can learn the ropes and identify problems, e.g. collecting samples, centrifuging and getting them appropriately stored. Make sure all equipment required is available.

When can you do it?

There is no point planning a study if you do not have the time to undertake it. An estimate of the amount of time that needs to be devoted to a particular study is paramount. This might involve protected time for one day a week or full-time research over a 2–3 year period. Trying to undertake a research project without adequate time is likely to lead to personal frustration, failure of the project and, ultimately, disillusionment from your supervisor or collaborators. If your current post is not a full-time research position, you will need to barter with your employer for protected time or try to conduct the research in your own time. If the clinical research project involves the use of a piece of laboratory equipment on a regular basis, you will not be able to complete the study if you are pulled away to an out-patient clinic to cover others. Negotiated protected time is paramount. Finally, remember, it always takes longer to complete a study than anticipated.

Is it of interest?

Is the research you are planning of interest to you and is it of interest to others? There is no point venturing into a research project if your heart is not in it and the subject matter does not stimulate you. You will rapidly become disillusioned and will not complete the study. Equally, the research project has to be of interest to others, particularly if you plan to try to present your findings at a clinical meeting or publish the results. The novice researcher will need to rely on a supervisor or colleague to point them in the right direction. A detailed search of the literature may bring to light a new slant to a particular planned research project which is topical and can be easily incorporated into the protocol at the planning stage. Alternatively, you may find out that the project in question has been done before and has been recently published. It is also worth discussing the planned research project with other colleagues or researchers, especially those with an interest in the particular field in question. Such discussion at an early stage will identify possible shortcomings, other people to speak to and the techniques that might be required.

Choice of Collaborators

It is critical to choose one's collaborators on the basis of their capacity to contribute essential ingredients to the project. Most projects these days require a multitude of partners, and each partner should bring a different perspective of expertise to the problem, e.g. recruitment potential, data analysis skills, clinical proficiency, etc. The multiple resources of the various collaborators not only ensure that the project will move toward completion, but also that the issue is not narrowly defined or interrupted.

Will collaborators be required?

Most research projects require the participation of a team of experts from various areas. An expert collaborator may be a statistician, pathologist, clinical chemist, or technician within a laboratory. Statisticians are possibly the most frequent collaborators because reliable interpretation of the data collated is paramount.

Data collection, documentation and useful tips

All paperwork and documentation is important. Keep up to date and write legibly. Using a notebook to document methods, results and deviations from the protocol is important. It is often necessary, at the end of a study, to find a vital piece of information and, if this has not been recorded, it may have been lost. The provision of a filing system which enables rapid access to patient records and other information, for example, the investigator protocol or procedures to be taken in the event of an adverse outcome, is essential. If you fail to record data or lose important information, you may incur the wrath of your supervisor. Furthermore, a mistake such as this will probably be remembered and mean you may not be invited to participate in other studies. If you are involved with a clinical study requiring intervention with a therapeutic agent, make yourself familiar with what to do if an adverse event occurs—whom to contact and the information that will be required. Attending at a course to enhance good clinical practice (GCP Diploma) will save time in the end. You must be contactable at all times in case of problems associated with your study, whether these are laboratory or clinical in nature; many problems can be averted by a simple telephone call. It is also advisable to try to make sure

focus on...
THE CLINICAL RESEARCH TEAM

Successful clinical research usually relies upon the coordinated activity of a large number of individuals. Of course, if you're conducting your own research project you may not have the luxury of such a level of support, but in a clinical trial a large team is assembled.

Not all trials or hospitals will have all of these, but the most common individuals involved in a trial are:

The Investigator—ultimately responsible for the conduct of a trial at the investigating site

The Research Nurse—responsible for much of the day-to-day activities in the trial, e.g. interviewing patients, recruiting, taking samples, entering data on the case report form, and general administrative duties

The Secretary—you're planning on doing all your own filing, photocopying, typing, mailing, archiving...?

The Study Site Coordinator—responsible for administration of the trial (often a research nurse will act as study site coordinator)

The Technician—someone has to analyze patient samples

The Pharmacist—in drug trials the investigational product will usually be stored in the hospital pharmacy. You will need to liaise with the pharmacist regarding randomization codes (to ensure appropriate allocation of product to patients) and general availability. Were you anticipating holding study clinics outside working hours? Well, you'd better let your pharmacist know (and make it worth his/her while!)

The Clinical Trials Monitor—your point of contact with the sponsor. The monitor is a valuable source of practical advice on all aspects of participating in a clinical trial. When working with a team you need to ensure that everyone is functioning efficiently. You need to work hard to keep all team members motivated. You also need to plan for the almost inevitable absences of key members of the team, and ensure that someone else is available to perform their duties. In some trials, the sponsor may provide funds for some of the above (e.g. provision of a study site coordinator).

that someone else is familiar with the study and can stand in during periods of annual or sick leave.

Writing a research protocol

Writing a detailed research protocol is essential; it will help you to decide the aims and objectives of the study, what measurements need to be made, the group of patients to be studied and how the data will be analyzed. The final product should be clear and provide enough details for all those involved in the study, and will be required for submission to an ethics committee or to a funding organization for a research grant. Many funding organizations provide their own application forms with the relevant sections that need completing.

---

focus on...

THE PROTOCOL

WHAT IS IT?

The clinical protocol describes what the trial is seeking to achieve and how it intends to achieve it. The protocol provides information on the design and methodology, for example the inclusion and exclusion criteria. A clear, well thought out, well-written protocol is key to a successful clinical trial.

Once a protocol has been approved, it is essential that the clinical trial is carried out in accordance with this document.

Format of a research protocol
Background

This section details the clinical or scientific background in the research questionnaire. It might include information about the importance of the research, for example the prevalence of a particular condition in the population or the associated morbidity and mortality of that condition. It should be up to date with the literature, providing an overview of previous studies that relate to the research area and their relevance to the research plan. This will enable any person who is unfamiliar with the subject to develop a clear understanding of how the proposed study links with the current state of knowledge. The background section does not need to be an exhaustive overview of the subject matter, but should make it clear why further research needs to be done within this particular area.

Aim of the study

This section should be brief and set out exactly what the research project intends to investigate. Listing too many aims is unlikely to inspire confidence and it is best to limit the number of objectives to two or three. After developing a research protocol, the aims and objectives often become more focused.

Unrealistic Inclusion Criteria

Karen Bowen, Senior Clinical Research Coordinator, Kentucky Center for Clinical Research and Investigator Services, University of Kentucky Medical Center, Lexington, KY 40536-0305, USA

The decision to place clinical research studies at particular research sites is based upon several different factors including, but not limited to, the past research experience of the clinical investigator, the ability to recruit the needed study subjects, the geographic location, the number of competing studies and the working relationships between the study site and the study sponsor. Recently, we were invited to participate in a Phase II pharmacokinetic study which was looking at the spinal fluid levels of an investigational antibiotic. The medical monitor of the project was a long-time acquaintance of the principal investigator at our academic medical center. Upon this personal request, the principal investigator readily agreed to participate in the study which, on the surface, appeared to be fairly simple and straightforward—recruit patients who were scheduled to undergo a lumbar puncture for diagnostic purposes, obtain informed consent to administer one dose of an antibiotic and subsequently collect one extra sample of spinal fluid for pharmacokinetic testing. It did not take long to realize that one of the protocol exclusion criteria made it nearly impossible to recruit potential subjects; to meet the required body surface area, an individual had to be 85 lbs (38.5 kg) or less and needed to be an amputee! This was the only possible way that an adult would meet the strict, unrealistic inclusion criteria. Needless to say, the study was closed nationally with only four subjects enrolled. Those four subjects were enrolled from our site because of our affiliation with a Veterans Affairs Medical Center. The moral of the story is to carefully read and scrutinize the inclusion/exclusion criteria of a potential study and determine its feasibility before committing to the research. By following this easy advice, the time and effort of the principal investigator and the clinical research staff will be focused where it will reap the most benefit.

Having too many aims and objectives is likely to suggest that the project is over ambitious and, if submitted for research funding, is unlikely to be successful.

Plan of investigation

This section outlines the research project in detail and includes information about the research method to be used, for example a case-control study, a placebo-controlled clinical trial or a laboratory-based study. There are many different methods of collating research data, including prospectively (as the patients are identified), retrospectively (using known patients or previously recorded data) and cross-sectionally (taking a group of patients at a particular moment in time). It should also be made clear whether the study involves a placebo and/or is blinded to both subjects and researchers. The subjects under investigation should be described in detail, including information about where they will be recruited from. The

---

focus on...
RECRUITMENT

DID YOU KNOW?

Poor recruitment is a frequent problem in clinical trials. Part of the problem can certainly be laid at the door of the sponsor (e.g. too restrictive exclusion criteria) but more often than not it is due to failings on the part of the investigator. According to 1999 data, approximately 10% of centers participating in recent Pharmacia & Upjohn clinical trials recruited zero patients and another 10% managed to recruit only one!

PREDICTING NUMBERS

An investigator's estimate of potentially eligible patients determines the recruitment target assigned by the sponsor. There are many sources of information available to guide such estimates, and it is important to use as many as possible—since each has some failings. The sources used will also depend on whether the trial is in the acute or the chronic setting. The various sources of information on

eligibility include historical controls, databases and patient records. You should also consult colleagues and liaise with local hospitals with a view to pooling resources.

HOW TO RECRUIT?

Develop a strategy, and prepare to be flexible. You need to target your patient population as effectively as possible within the constraints of the finite resources you have at your disposal. Advertising may be appropriate—you need to consider where and when to advertise and ensure that any advertisements are approved by your local ethics committee. Networking with colleagues and local hospitals may also provide a sizeable referral volume.

WHEN TO RECRUIT?

You're not just being asked to recruit patients, you have to recruit them in a timely manner: the trial duration is finite. So, you need to plan early. If you fail to meet your recruitment target then you're unlikely to be invited to participate again – be it by the sponsor or a colleague – so it is in your interest to work hard at recruitment.

inclusion and exclusion criteria should be listed; this may involve restricting recruitment to patients of a certain age, sex, particular disease or complication, or current medication. An indication of the likely ease or difficulty in identifying these subjects should be made, for example the number of patients

---

Read the Small Print

Dr Charles Laurito, Associate Professor and Director of Pain,
Department of Anesthesiology, University of Illinois, Chicago, IL 60612, USA

We were approached by a pharmaceutical company and asked to help evaluate a novel therapy for pain management. The active agent being tested was unusual because it remained in suspension and had physical characteristics that, theoretically, provided months of pain relief following one epidural dosing. It had a very low pKa of 1.5, was highly lipid-soluble and tended to aggregate with itself. The patients who were eligible for the medication had to have disseminated cancers, suffer from pain despite the use of at least 40 mg of morphine sulfate per day, and have no disease spread that would preclude the use of an epidural injection. To be eligible, the patient also had to have a life expectancy of less than 6 months. The protocol was very complicated and detailed. The epidural was to be placed at a level as far cephalad as T4. Correct placement was confirmed with an Omnipaque injection to outline the epidural space and up to 5 mL of 2% lidocaine was injected slowly to alleviate the patient's most intense pain. Once this was documented, the patient received one of four different doses of the experimental medication. Since the active ingredient aggregated, 3 mL doses of the substance were alternated with 3 mL of normal saline until the entire dose was injected into the epidural space. Once the therapy was available, many of our patients felt an urgency to receive it because they wanted to try this new form of therapy. Even those who received adequate pain relief with opioid wanted to try a therapy that wouldn't have the side effects that morphine gave them. Almost all hoped they could decrease their doses of morphine. Since the medication could be injected only after epidural placement and confirmation with fluoroscopy, there was a lot of pressure for everything to work perfectly. With our first patient, we overstaffed the clinic with people who wanted to learn the protocol and lend a hand. The epidural needle and catheter were advanced easily, placement was confirmed with the contrast agent and fluoroscopy, and the medication was injected into the epidural space. A problem immediately developed in that once the first bolus was given, we were unable to flush with 3 mL of normal saline. After several attempts, the catheter was removed to show that the material had formed a solid mass within it. We were unable to dislodge this clot, despite tremendous pressures applied to the plungers of very small syringes. It was like concrete. We went back to the protocol and read it closely. The patient was discharged and the company's senior scientists contacted. After many hours of study, we discovered that we were using an epidural catheter made of a polyamide instead of the nylon catheters that had been used in the pre-clinical studies. The active agent, in the presence of Omnipaque, seemed to react with one, and not the other catheter to form a concrete aggregate. Once the change was discovered, we were able to bring the patient, and subsequent patients, in for successful treatment.

---

with a particular condition attending your clinic and the potential number of possible subjects from this number might be calculated. There is no point trying to recruit extremely rare cases in a single-center study, but it might be possible to recruit the required number using multiple centers. An indication of how the patients will be identified should be made—many clinical services now employ clinical information workstations where details about patients and their problems are readily accessible. For some conditions, this might require recruitment from primary care, for example a clinical study involving patients with Type 2 diabetes who are diet controlled may not be possible if confined to secondary care since most of these patients are managed in primary care. Going through this process of identifying and determining the potential number of subjects will reap benefits in the long term. If the subjects

Creative Recruiting

Robert Segraves, Department of Psychiatry, Case Western Reserve University School of Medicine, and MetroHealth Medical Center, Cleveland, OH 44109-1998, USA

Rapid recruitment of subjects for a clinical trial can often make or break a project. We recently conducted a trial on the pharmacological treatment of premature ejaculation. Unfortunately, other sites in our area were also recruiting subjects for trials with similar indications and we had considerable trouble locating sufficient subjects. Several local radio stations refused to run our advertisements because they were afraid that male listeners would be offended. Furthermore, our newspaper advertising budget was almost gone and we still needed more subjects. I was tempted to concede defeat. Instead, my coordinator and I reviewed the strategy of other centers, analyzed our efforts to date and decided on ways to both maximize our current recruitment efforts and reach alternative audiences. First, we realized that most men responding to the newspaper advertisement refused to leave their contact telephone number because they feared that one of their work colleagues would find out what they had done. Our advertisements were, therefore, changed to specify certain hours of the day when the coordinator was available to answer calls. Second, we realized that we had neglected to place our advertisements where potential subjects would read them. Thus, we moved them from the Sunday medical section of the local paper to the daily sports section on days after games played by local sports teams. Third, we realized that no one had advertised in any of the newspapers targeting homosexual men. We, therefore, placed advertisements in newspapers featuring alternative lifestyles. As a result of these changes, we reached our recruitment goal. The moral of the story is to stop when current strategies are not working, review the strategy and think of ways to both maximize recruitment and reach new audiences.

cannot be recruited, the study will fail and is very unlikely to get funding from national organizations.

The data to be collected should be listed. An indication of who will collect these data and how they will be analyzed should be made. The development of a proforma to be used by the researcher will often save time in the long term as it is less likely that essential data will be missed or not collected. Details of how the measurements are to be made should be included—

focus on...
ESSENTIAL AND SOURCE DOCUMENTS

WHAT ARE THEY?
What the trial is seeking to achieve and how it intends to achieve it are described in the clinical protocol. The protocol provides information on the design and methodology, for example the inclusion and exclusion criteria. A clear, well thought out, well-written protocol is key to a successful clinical trial. Once a protocol has been approved, it is essential that the clinical trial is carried out in accordance with that document. In the context of regular quality assurance checks during a clinical trial, ensuring that data are accurately recorded and transcribed is essential. Source data verification refers to the procedure whereby a clinical trial monitor directly compares data written in the case report form (CRF) with that contained within the source documents (e.g. patient files). Often source data verification will be carried out during a study. This is a lengthy procedure and it is therefore important that you arrange for a suitable room for the monitor and that all relevant documentation is available. What are they? A common cause of confusion, the distinction

between source documents and essential documents is reasonably clear cut (although occasionally there is overlap, with some documents being both source and essential).

ESSENTIAL DOCUMENTS
According to ICH-GCP, essential documents are those which: "Individually and collectively permit evaluation of the conduct of a trial and the quality of the data produced. These documents serve to demonstrate the compliance of the investigator, sponsor and monitor with the standards of good clinical practice and with all applicable regulatory requirements". Fundamentally, essential documents are trial-specific documents —the investigator's brochure, a signed copy of the protocol, a sample CRF, the informed consent form, advertisements for subject recruitment....

The ICH-GCP provides a minimum list of essential documents—there are 53 categories!

SOURCE DOCUMENTS
Don't be fooled by the 'essential' in essential documents—source documents are also 'essential'. Source documents are the original data and records relating to particular patients—hospital records, X-rays, pharmacy records, i.e. the source of the data entered on the CRF.

when the subject is studied, how blood samples are taken, how blood pressure is measured, etc. An indication of where the subjects will be studied should be described. Will this be under laboratory conditions or will they be out-patients? Who will perform the different parts of the study? In those studies where subjects are randomized or the treatment is either a placebo or active drug, an indication of the method of randomization should be described and an estimate of the sample size required to obtain a significant result should be calculated. Without this estimate, the study may be too small to provide conclusive data about the research question under investigation. Furthermore, it makes it less likely that the research will be published. Involvement of a statistician may be required at this stage.

Ethical issues

Ethical issues should also be discussed. An application will need to be forwarded to your local research ethics committee for approval to undertake research in either volunteers or patients. The role of this body is two-fold:

- to protect the subjects from potentially harmful or frankly dangerous practices

- to protect the researcher from possible future legal difficulties

Most research ethics committees consist of academics, medical doctors, nursing staff and lay people. Many funding organizations will require confirmation before releasing funds.

Justification for support and facilities available

A detailed breakdown of how the funds will be used is of the highest importance. These figures need to be accurate, as those reading the proposal will be familiar with costings. The locations where the research will take place and existing items of equipment that may be used in the study need to be listed.

References

At the end of the research plan the references should be detailed and reflect up-to-date papers.

Clinical trial design

Many studies involve the use of a therapeutic drug, either as part of an in-house single-center clinical study or as part of a multi-center study. A team of experts who have formulated the trial design in order to answer a particular question coordinate most large multi-center studies. This type of intervention trial is usually stimulated by a pharmaceutical institution developing a novel agent and involves collaboration with these experts. By the time the novel agent is given to human volunteers or patients, it has usually been extensively studied in the laboratory and in experimental animal models. Clinical trials of novel therapeutic agents are an important area of research since potential problems or adverse effects often do not come to light until this stage. It is important that all adverse side effects are taken seriously and documented.

The terminology of the trial design can be confusing to a novice researcher. Initial studies using a novel agent tend to be open or uncontrolled studies to allow determination of whether an agent is effective and what doses are needed to produce a therapeutic response (efficacy). Trials at this stage will also shed light on how well or badly the drug is tolerated (tolerability). In these types of study design, both patients and researcher know exactly what is administered (hence, 'open') and the novel agent is not compared to anything else (hence, 'uncontrolled'). Open and uncontrolled studies allow dose-response data to be obtained. Thus, a new agent may be given to subjects at differing doses to assess whether it influences the frequency or severity of the condition under investigation. Although this type of trial design may under- or over-estimate the potential for this new agent, it is a prerequisite step before proceeding to more demanding controlled trials.

In controlled trials, the efficacy of a new drug is compared in a head-to-head manner with either a placebo or a standard treatment option currently in clinical use. In a single-blind study, the volunteer or patient does not know what treatment is being taken, but the researcher or doctor does. This study design is

focus on...

CLINICAL TRIAL DESIGN

If you are participating in a sponsored trial then the design of the trial will have been predetermined, and all you need to know is how to implement the design (e.g. how to assign randomization codes). If you are thinking of setting up your own trial then there's no substitute for talking to colleagues and reading up as widely as possible.

The most important issue is to come up with a good question and to formulate a hypothesis based on this question. Assuming that it is a reasonable hypothesis the problem then becomes one of hypothesis testing— what is the best way of determining whether your hypothesis is true (from a statistical standpoint) or false.

Important aspects of clinical trial design include:

CONTROLS

Trials will often be comparing different treatments or interventions. The control group provides a basis against which results in the treatment groups can be compared. Controls can be active— generally 'standard of care'—or inactive (placebo). Sometimes so-called historical controls are used—using data from previous trials as the control. Since few trials are identical in design and patient population, such comparisons should be avoided where possible.

RANDOMIZATION

This is the process of randomly allocating patients to each arm of the study in an attempt to ensure that the groups are as similar as possible such that the results can be attributed only to chance or to the therapeutic intervention— i.e. to eliminate potential bias.

BLINDING

This is the process of ensuring that various participants in the trial are unaware of which treatment groups the subjects are in. In single-blind trials, the subject is unaware of what treatment he/she is receiving; in double-blind trials, both subject and investigator are unaware of which treatment the subject is receiving. Single-blind trials run the risk of the investigator behaving differently towards subjects in each group— i.e. there is potentially a management bias that could adversely affect interpretation of the study.

PARALLEL AND CROSSOVER STUDIES

In parallel-group studies, each group (control and treatment) receives only one treatment for the whole trial; in crossover studies, each group receives both treatments (after a suitable washout period after the first part of the trial). The disadvantages of a crossover design are primarily the length (twice as long at least as an equivalent parallel-group study) and the fact that the first treatment is likely to have affected the condition in some way affording a potentially different baseline state at the start of the second treatment.

essential for finding out whether the treatment dose has to be titrated to achieve the desired result and the sort of side effects to expect. Nonetheless, in a single-blind study there is the potential for observer bias to influence the assessment or recording of the data. Double-blind studies offer the best chance of eliminating bias since both the subject under observation and the researcher are both ignorant of the therapy under question.

Many trials use a comparative group or a crossover design. In comparative studies, there are two or more groups receiving differing therapies, with one of the groups receiving the novel agent under investigation. These trials require many subjects or patients and it may not be easy to recruit into this type of study. Furthermore, it has to be assumed that each group of patients behave in the same manner. This shortcoming can be overcome in a crossover trial; the groups under observation receive all the treatments, generally in a random order. In this type of trial, all the patients behave as their own control. Crossover trials are suitable for chronic conditions, for example diabetes. Thus, a group of patients may be treated with one type of oral hypoglycemic agent and subsequently with a novel oral hypoglycemic agent. However, there are potential problems, in

focus on...

RESPONSIBILITIES OF THE INVESTIGATOR

Although many of the duties in a trial are undertaken by other members of staff, the investigator is responsible for the overall conduct of a clinical trial at the investigating site. The primary responsibilities of an investigator are:

- to ensure that sufficient resources (patients, personnel, equipment, space and time) are available for the duration of the trial

- to submit the protocol and related information (e.g. informed consent form) to the local ethics committee for approval

- to obtain informed consent from all subjects taking part in the trial

- to document all data appropriately

- to inform the sponsor and, where necessary, the ethics committee of the occurrence of all serious adverse events

- to be available and to make all necessary data, paperwork and personnel available for source data verification, audit or inspection purposes

- to sign off on the study report

- to archive all data following the completion of the trial for the agreed time period

It is certainly worth reading all the paperwork closely and researching appropriately before agreeing to participate in a trial. It is in no one's interests for you to fall short on any of these.

that there may be an order effect; it is possible that the first therapeutic agent may dramatically improve the condition or the effects of the first agent may persist and overlap with the effects of the second treatment.

Compliance is an important issue in clinical trials. Failure to respond to a particular therapy may be due to the subject simply forgetting to take the tablets, whether intentional or not. Therefore, in any intervention trial it is important to assess compliance with therapy, in order to be certain that a drug failure is not simply due to non-compliance. The most effective

Advice from a Clinical Trials Coordinator

Erin A Spousta, RN, BSN, Clinical Research Coordinator, Coronary and Peripheral Interventions, Austin Heart Institute, 4600 Seton Center Parkway, #816, Austin, TX 78759-5258, USA

I think my most difficult trial in terms of recruitment and eligibility is an ongoing angiogenesis trial for intermittent claudication. The selection criteria are so tight that I have to screen 7–12 patients just to find one who is eligible. The main exclusion criterion is any evidence of cancer, and the patients who are interested in the trial must go through extensive cancer screening to determine their eligibility, as well as complete two exercise treadmill tests (>1 minute and <12 minutes) with their main reason for stopping being severe pain in their legs and nothing else.

I have run ads and submitted press releases about dosing our first patient in the local papers, hoping that this would spark some interest among potential candidates. I have placed posters in the waiting room of the only vascular surgeon (in town) as well as the office of a local radiology group in attempts to attract patients. We are trying to get the local news media in for an interview about the trial so that people will see it on television. I have even gone as far as having our medical records department run diagnosis codes to get the names of all the patients we care for with the diagnosis of intermittent claudication or peripheral vascular disease; I have started to screen the patient charts.

The moral of the story is that the clinical trials coordinator needs to be creative with recruitment. Pull diagnosis codes, put ads in papers, talk to physicians in other offices about finding potential candidates in their practice for referral to the trial, hang posters in hospital or medical office elevators—anything to catch the potential patient's attention and interest. Most importantly, get the principal investigator to speak to a potential patient about the trial before you, as the coordinator, speak to them regarding their interest with a view to obtaining informed consent. Patients really tend to respond well if they hear about a trial from a physician and get their opinion as to whether or not they should participate.

approach for reducing non-compliance is to anticipate and to spend time instructing the subjects or patients carefully and frequently with this in mind.

Clinical Research in a Private Practice Environment

Dr James Ferguson, Baylor College of Medicine, St Luke's Episcopal Hospital, Texas Heart Institute, Houston, USA

One of the most important lessons we learnt while putting together the Cardiology Research Department at the Texas Heart Institute was 'neutrality'. Unlike many institutions which have traditional monolithic cardiology sections, cardiology at St Luke's Episcopal Hospital and the Texas Heart Institute is actually an amalgam of a number of small to medium sized cardiology groups. In this sort of multilateral environment, research has previously been handicapped by the political difficulties of inter-group competition.

When I came to the Texas Heart Institute in 1987, I had the good fortune of teaming up with Mary Harlan, a very experienced research coordinator who knew all too well the complexities of the system and the internal politics. We established a Cardiology Research Department that was neutral, that was apolitical and that did not compete with the individual cardiology groups. We made a conscious effort not to favor any one group and gave all the groups and all the physicians an opportunity to participate in the protocols. Yes, we did favor those willing to work with us, but what we ultimately created was one of the few truly unified aspects in cardiology. We also forged close ties with the hospital and, rather being positioned as adversaries, work closely with the administrators of St Luke's Hospital to select protocols that are clinically relevant without draining the institutional financial resources. The end result is shown below.

The Cardiology Research Department is a central 'neutral' resource that facilitates clinical research by practicing physicians at St Luke's under the umbrella of the Texas Heart Institute. We provide these physicians with capabilities that they would not otherwise have, such as protocol and consent writing, data collection, data handling, and Institutional Review Board and sponsor interaction. By providing tangible benefit, and by not playing political favorites, we have become a true central resource that is efficient, capable and attractive to potential sponsors. The practicing physicians serve as primary investigators, and if this requires substantial time commitments, are compensated for their time and effort.

The key to success in a busy clinical institution, such as ours, is an open environment. Our physicians have quickly recognized that clinical research is more than just onerous drudgery: it is a chance to really advance the standard of care in a meaningful way. Rather than having them work for us, we work for them and the end result benefits everyone. On a bulletin board above my desk I have posted an anonymous quotation that I firmly adhere to: "there is no limit on what you can accomplish if you don't insist on taking credit for it". Clinical research in a private practice environment is a perfect example of that.

Conclusion

Entering research can be a daunting period. However, the benefits of undertaking research are great; it will not only stimulate your mind but is likely to further your career.

Further reading

Lloyd J, Raven A, editors. Handbook of clinical research. London: Churchill Medical Communications, 1994.

CHAPTER 5
Transforming ideas into research

David Rowland & James Thornton

In order for research to be valuable, the data must yield reasonably clear and meaningful results. Guaranteeing such endpoints is never possible, but carrying out a poorly designed project will almost always produce 'garbage' results that are generally uninterpretable. Numerous worthwhile projects have come to naught because investigators have not taken the time to think through the details of the study before carrying it out. Even with a well-designed study that yields clear findings, investigators need to know the limitations inherent in the research process, as well as in the specific research designs and protocols they use.

This chapter is intended to help the investigator understand the process of transforming empirical questions into procedures that improve the likelihood of reaching confident data-based conclusions. Without some understanding and appreciation of the research process, a potential investigator may not know whether he/she possesses the basic knowledge, skills and resources to carry out research effectively, or even whether he/she values the research process sufficiently to invest his/her time and energy.

A critical **first** step in this process involves asking basic questions about the research design and protocol to ensure that the study procedures adequately match the research objectives. Such questions must address every detail of the project, from beginning to end, with most good research projects anticipating the specific kinds of data analysis, results and probable conclusions long before the first piece of data has even been collected. Although this chapter provides only limited explanations to such questions, investigators who are at least cognizant of these questions are likely to design a better project.

Key Elements in the Research Process

- establishing research hypotheses
- defining and measuring variables
- collecting data
- statistical analysis and hypothesis testing
- drawing conclusions

What are the research questions?

At the beginning of every research project is a list of questions, usually referred to as research hypotheses, that the study intends to address. These research hypotheses are often ordered into levels of importance. In some instances, they represent specific applications of larger, more general theories (i.e. general to specific, a deductive process); in others, they represent specific tests carried out on samples for the purpose of generalizing to broader populations (i.e. specific to general, an inductive process). Most research programs involve combinations of these processes, with theories spawning new hypotheses, and/or the results of hypothesis testing shaping new ideas and theories.

Perhaps more relevant to this discussion, embedded within every research hypothesis are the variables that become the crux of the study. In most research, one or several variables are designated outcome or dependent—the variables the investigator is interested in measuring or understanding. The other variables are usually predictor or independent (also treatment)—the variables suspected of affecting the outcome variables. For example, in the hypothesis, 'a diet low in saturated fats improves cardiovascular health', cardiovascular health is the outcome or dependent variable which is presumed to be affected by a certain type of diet—the predictor or independent variable. This simple hypothesis might be elaborated by introducing a second independent variable, 'a diet low in saturated fats combined with exercise improves cardiovascular health'. Multiple endpoints can also be added by stating, 'a diet low in saturated fats reduces arterial plaques, which improves cardiovascular health'. In this last statement, an intervening variable, arterial plaques, has been introduced to explain the effects of the diet on cardiovascular health.

Although each of these statements appear to be simple enough, each calls for a different type of research design and, subsequently, a different statistical analysis.

Knowing the nature of your variables

Once the hypotheses have been formulated, familiarity with the study variables and knowing how they will eventually be defined becomes a critical **second** step in the research process. Important not only to the research process, this step will also help the investigator determine whether he/she has access to the necessary resources (e.g. basic equipment or personnel to score psychometric tests) to carry out the study.

Variables must first be defined procedurally with an operational definition before the relationship between them can be studied. This is one of the most critical steps in the research preparation process, yet it is often overlooked as a simple or self-evident process. Projects sometimes suffer because investigators choose measures that are not widely accepted or are even inappropriate for the research questions they are asking. For example, if cardiovascular health is being investigated, is it assessed with blood pressure, heart rate, heart stroke volume, arterial patency, plasma cholesterol or some other measure? Should assessments be taken during a physical challenge or in a resting state? Also, how might all these measures be interrelated? Often no single definition is completely satisfactory, so the key is to begin with previous research published in well-known journals that relies on existing or standardized measures acceptable to the field. Such definitions can often provide a foundation for the study's measures, which can then be elaborated in order to address the specific goals of the study at hand. In using such a strategy, the investigator can cite successful studies using similar definitions, while simultaneously building the knowledge base of the field.

This same process of defining variables needs to be applied to all the variables under investigation, including independent variables. For example, how is a diet low in saturated fats, an effective dose of a drug, or a treatment with cognitive-behavioral therapy to be defined?

How sophisticated do the outcome measures need to be?

The answer to this question depends on a number of factors, including the outcome variable under investigation and the conventions for the particular area of research. One common strategy is to choose more sensitive measures (assuming they are available) over less sensitive ones. A measure that ends up being overly sensitive can be reduced to lesser sensitivity; the opposite does not hold.

Sensitivity refers to the ability of the outcome measure to detect changes, a characteristic that partly depends on the scale of measurement. In some instances, the outcome measure need not be particularly sensitive or refined, and might represent a simple 'yes' or 'no' categorization (referred to as a categorical or nominal variable). Did the patient die? Did the woman become pregnant? Did the child contract the disease? However, more often than not, yes or no outcomes represent endpoints along a continuum. For example, in answer to the question 'did the child recover function of his limb?' the possible responses might be ordered from 'no' to 'mild improvement' to 'great improvement' to 'complete recovery'. The categorical yes/no variable has now been transformed into an ordinal scale of improvement that yields more sensitive information. While such ratings may reflect global subjective judgments on the part of the clinician, they are most useful when they are based on more objective criteria derived from continuously scaled interval or ratio measures. Elaborating on our present example, a subjective global judgment based on such measures as 'the range of arm movement measured in decimeters', 'muscle flexion capability' and 'sensory thresholds' establishes an objective basis for a global judgment. These interval or ratio measures are very precise and yield numbers that have clearly defined relationships with one another. For example, the investigator can know precisely how a range of 20 decimeters of limb movement compares with a range of 15 decimeters. However, he/she cannot be sure how 'great improvement' compares with 'mild improvement', other than to state that the former represents the more desirable outcome.

Usually a movement from nominal to ordinal to interval/ratio scales of measurement (with the latter scales representing the 'higher' levels of measurement) can be thought of as a progression in sensitivity and refinement. In general, the higher the scale or level of measurement, the more assumptions can be made about the relationships of the numbers to each other in the data set, as well as about the general distribution of those numbers. Because of these characteristics, statistical analyses will be more able to detect a relationship between the outcome and the independent variables when the researcher uses a higher level of measurement. Stated slightly differently, use of a higher scale means the investigator will be less likely to err by missing an effect that really exists between the variables in the population (this type of error is discussed in considerable detail later in this chapter).

Although interval/ratio measures often improve objectivity and sensitivity, they sometimes have the disadvantage of being less relevant from a clinical standpoint. An improvement in range of limb movement from 0–30 decimeters may be statistically significant, but conveys little information regarding the recovery of functional use of the limb. In contrast, a global judgment such as 'near complete' recovery may provide extremely useful clinical information. The challenge is one of using objective and sensitive outcome measures, yet identifying endpoints that are also clinically relevant. A pertinent example can be seen in the research on 'sexual satisfaction' in men using a pharmacological treatment for erectile failure. Improvements in erectile capacity (e.g. measured in terms of mm increase in penile circumference) impart little benefit if they do produce sufficient rigidity to enable vaginal intromission. One way to approach this dilemma is to collect as sensitive data as possible using interval or ratio-scaled variables, then construct ordinal categories or dichotomous outcomes from them. For example, the investigator might decide that any increase in penile circumference greater than 20 mm is clinically significant, since most men can achieve intromission under such conditions. Alternatively, he/she might incorporate additional endpoints into the project, for example, whether the man is able to achieve vaginal penetration (a reasonably objective yes-no dichotomy) and how satisfied the man is with his erectile capacity (an important subjective measure that can be ordinally scaled from 'none' to 'complete'). Ultimately, the issue needs to be resolved by the investigators themselves as they consider the goals of their project and the audience they are targeting.

Assuming multiple measures for the outcome variable, which one(s) should the investigator ultimately use?

In generating multiple measures for the outcome variable, the investigator is more likely to ensure that an important outcome measure is not omitted, as well as to address issues of objectivity, sensitivity and clinical relevance.

Since most research constructs such as 'cardiovascular health' and 'sexual satisfaction' represent constellations of behavioral or physiological responses, often their definition defies a simple, single measure outcome. It is equally likely that there may be no single accepted definition for the construct. In such instances, the investigator may decide to develop an index or composite that represents several measures simultaneously. Such indices may be derived from a combination of variables of differing levels of measurement (nominal, ordinal, interval), but each usually must first be reduced to the scale of the least refined measure. Using the example of sexual satisfaction, the investigator might construct a summary index indicating overall amount of 'improvement' based on three measures, with each being transformed to a simple dichotomous outcome such that 'improvement' = 1 and 'no improvement' = 0. These three measures might include:

- a 20 mm or greater increase in penile circumference

- the ability to achieve vaginal intromission

- the patient's indication of at least partial satisfaction of erectile function based on a subjective 4-point scale ranging from 'none' to 'complete'

The outcome variable now incorporates three components related to the construct and can be represented by an ordered 4-point scale ranging from 0–3.

Such indices can be highly useful for developing clinically relevant endpoints, but they come with important caveats. The investigator usually must provide *a priori* rationales for cutoff points that transform the continuous or ordinal variables to simple dichotomous outcomes. Second, the individual measures should not be assessing essentially identical things (this would inflate outcome differences among individuals), although each measure should be relevant to the overall endpoint. Finally, the investigator will have to decide whether to weight the measures equally, or to assign greater weights to specific measures on the assumption that they contribute more to the definition of the construct. These procedures are sometimes risky for new investigators entering the field, as such cutoffs and weighting often generate significant controversy and may easily become a target of criticism by reviewers [1].

Critical questions summarized

When considering the nature of the variables, the investigator should take into consideration the following questions:

- how will each variable be defined and measured?

- are there standardized or existing measures that can be used?

- are the resources available to apply these measures?

- how satisfactory are the existing measures?

- what level of sophistication and sensitivity can be achieved and/or is appropriate?

- how objective do the measures need to be?

- how important is it to have clinically relevant measures?

- will multiple measures be required for the outcome variable?

- will it be necessary to construct indices or composites from multiple measures?

Collecting and Managing Data

Although some clinical research may utilize data sets drawn from existing data banks, most involve active data collection. Data collection entails the ancillary responsibilities of data organization and storage. As easy as this might sound, these processes typically require resources beyond existing office personnel. Most clinical studies of any size employ a records keeper or data manager. This individual ensures that data collection proceeds properly and meticulously, and that the data are organized and coded in a timely manner with sufficient documentation so they can be understood long after his/her departure. In addition, this person may need to transcribe the data before entering them into a data file, a process which itself may necessitate dedicated computer hardware and software. Storage of hardcopy records may require substantial filing space. In all, the process of data management is likely to entail significant investments of staff time as well as some capital expense.

While the data manager assumes responsibility for detailed oversight of data and data files, the project director should take a hands-on approach with the data as well, though at a different level. Without breaking blinding codes, the project director should periodically (more often at the outset of the study) review data records to ascertain that data values are falling within expected ranges, that unusual values or patterns are investigated and understood, and that subsequent modifications to the protocol are implemented as quickly as possible.

The logic behind hypothesis testing

Hypothesis testing is the essential power tool of the empirical investigator, and understanding this process and its limitations is critical for any clinician considering substantial involvement in a research endeavor.

Testing the null hypothesis

Underlying every research question or hypothesis suggesting a relationship between two or more variables is a statement of the opposite (usually negated) condition or outcome. This statement, called the null hypothesis, actually states that any change or variation in the outcome variable is the result of chance (as opposed to the independent variable). The null hypothesis serves an important function in that it is the only hypothesis in the study that can be tested directly.

Why? In a nutshell, every outcome measure (e.g. cardiovascular health) shows random variation, both among individuals and within individuals over time (called measurement error). The goal of most research is to demonstrate relationships between (or among) variables, i.e. to show that variation in the outcome variable is related to variation in independent variables. But variation in the outcome variable can never exclusively be attributed to the independent variable (as our research hypothesis states) since some of this variation results from random fluctuation. For example, variation or change in cardiovascular health among participants results from:

- random variation (from sampling or measurement error)
- the independent variable—a diet low in saturated fats

Of course, the problem lies in the fact that the investigator never knows how much of the variation can be attributed to random fluctuation or chance (some of it? all of it?), and how much to the independent variable.

So scientific methodology requires that the null hypothesis be tested—this hypothesis states that any changes in the outcome variable are the result of chance and therefore by implication they are not related to the independent variable. Inferential statistical tests, the kind used in most analyses and which lead to conclusions of 'significance', allow the investigator to determine the probability that changes in the outcome variable occurred mainly from chance or random variation. If it is not likely that they occurred mainly by chance (usually considered as 1 out of 20 times or less, or ≤ 0.05), then the investigator invokes another variable, namely the independent variable, to explain the variation in the outcome variable. In research language, the investigator rejects the null hypothesis, and in doing so accepts the alternative research hypothesis, which states that variation in the outcome is related to the independent variable.

Thus, investigators either accept the null hypothesis or they reject it. In doing the latter, they turn to the research hypothesis as the next best explanation available. While this may sound confusing, it boils down to a simple process. If we believe (from statistical evidence) that the changes in the outcome are due to more than random fluctuation, then we are willing to attribute those changes to the independent variable. But as is now evident, acceptance of the research hypothesis does not result from testing it directly. That is, there is no direct evidence based on the scientific method that the independent variable is affecting the outcome variable. Our acceptance of the research hypothesis results from rejecting the competing null hypothesis. So why is it important to understand all this?

Design flaws and errors

Understanding the above process is critical for avoiding flaws in research design and minimizing errors leading to accepting the wrong hypothesis. There are several errors that can be made in the research process and each is discussed briefly below.

Confounding factors

It is sometimes said that a project has a 'fatal flaw'. Such flaws, which can lead to erroneous conclusions, refer to the fact that variables other than the independent variable (these other variables are called extraneous variables) are likely to be varying along with independent variables in the study. Therefore, to conclude that variation in the outcome measure is due exclusively, or even predominantly, to the independent variable cannot be justified. For example, a diet low in saturated fats might be accompanied by a tendency to increase intake of other food groups that are healthier and thus have the potential to lower cholesterol levels on their own. Therefore, unless diet is strictly regulated, not only in terms of saturated fats but also in other food groups, it will not be possible to make conclusions about the effect of lowered saturated fat intake on cardiovascular health. Such flaws represent problems in the design of the experiment, and lead to a condition known as confounding—a situation where the outcome of the study cannot be attributed exclusively to variation in the independent variables under investigation because other variables are changing simultaneously. Confounding greatly weakens the investigator's capacity to draw conclusions of any strength, and often leaves the investigator in the position of having to acknowledge a flaw that may render the findings inconclusive.

To avoid problems later, an important **third** step in preparing for a research project is to spend significant time and energy beforehand identifying possible extraneous variables that might confound the study. This process may require a review of similar studies on the topic as well as assuming a devil's advocate role regarding the tenability of any presumed (desired) relationship between independent and outcome variables. Once identified, these extraneous variables may be handled in a variety of ways. They might be held constant by the investigator (e.g. strictly regulating the diet of the participant). They might be controlled through a process of randomized assignment to treatment groups. They might be controlled through the sampling process (e.g. limiting the sample only to participants who consume high levels of saturated fat in their diet). Or they might simply be measured as part of the study so that any potential effect can be statistically controlled in the data analysis (e.g. requiring participants to keep daily records of their type and amount of food intake).

Each of the above strategies, though critical to the overall viability of a study, has disadvantages. For example, often it is not possible to hold an extraneous variable constant unless the study is carried out in a highly controlled (and often expensive) environment. True random assignment always has the potential to generate groups that are grossly unequal on relevant variables (e.g. sex or age of participants) at the outset of the study—a very undesirable situation. In sampling a subpopulation of participants with high-saturated-fat diets, the investigator may be limited in generalizing the research conclusions to the larger target population. In using statistical controls, the investigator sacrifices 'degrees of freedom' in the statistical analysis, making it more difficult to achieve a significant effect. In this last strategy, the loss of a single degree of freedom by statistically controlling one extraneous variable may have only limited impact on the conclusions of the study. If variation from a number of extraneous variables is controlled in this fashion, the resulting loss in degrees of freedom may have a substantial impact on the investigator's ability to accept the research hypothesis.

Nevertheless, the 'cost' of any of the procedures above for handling extraneous variables far outweighs the problems encountered when possible confounding variables have not been identified and adequately taken into account.

Making errors by accepting the incorrect hypothesis

The investigator never actually knows which hypothesis—the research or null—represents the true state of affairs in the population. Research conclusions are based upon the *likelihood* of one of the hypotheses being true. As such, any research conclusion is subject to error.

For example, the investigator may reject the null hypothesis when it is true. This error, known as a Type I error, means that the investigator has erroneously attributed variation in the outcome variable to the independent variable, when in fact the variation resulted simply from random fluctuation. This error might be viewed as an 'over-estimation' of the effect of the independent variable.

The probability of a Type I error, known as alpha (α), is easily quantified, as it is equal to the significance level selected by the investigator. Scientific convention generally sets this probability at 0.05 or 1 in 20, meaning that if the outcome occurs once out of 20 times or less by chance alone ($p \leq 0.05$) then the investigator attributes the variation to the independent variable. The α level is also known as the 'significance level', and this criterion must be met or exceeded in order to conclude a significant relationship between two or more variables.

How does the significance level represent the probability of a Type I error? Consider the following logic:

- whenever variation in the outcome occurs 1 out of 20 times or less ($p \leq 0.05$) from random fluctuation, the investigator will attribute the variation to the independent variable

- this amount of variation in the outcome variable can occur simply by chance (that is, 1 in 20 times or less) regardless of whether the independent variable was affecting the outcome variable

- each and every time the outcome occurs 1 out of 20 times or less by chance the investigator attributes the variation to the independent variable, therefore, on average, the investigator errs 1 out of 20 times in his/her conclusion

Stated in another way, it can be readily seen that if 20 studies were carried out and each yielded significant results at the 0.05 level, then the conclusion of one of them is likely to have been wrong. Although investigators can state precisely the probability of making a Type I error, unfortunately they never know in which specific situation or study they might have made that error.

An expedient way to decrease the probability of a Type I error is to change the significance level to something more stringent, say 0.01 or 0.001. This cannot be done without the consequence of increasing the likelihood of making a second type of error.

This second type of error, appropriately called a Type II error, occurs when the investigator accepts the null hypothesis when it is false, thereby rejecting the 'true' research hypothesis. This kind of error, perhaps akin to 'under-estimating' the effect of the independent variable, is not as easy to quantify, as its probability, known as beta (β), is affected by a number of factors. However, in general, β is related to how much 'noise' (unexplained or random variation known as error[1]) exists in the data, and more specifically, the ratio of:

$$\frac{\text{independent variable effect (explained variation)}}{\text{noise (unexplained variation or error)}}$$

The probability of a Type II error can be minimized by reducing noise or unexplained variation (the denominator), or by increasing the effect or variation in the independent variable (the numerator), or by doing both. Stated simply, the stronger the independent variable effect stands out against the background noise, the more likely the investigator will detect the effect.

The limits of hypothesis testing

Hypothesis testing never reveals which of our hypotheses—research or null—is true, but only which of the two is probably true. Because conclusions in science reflect probabilistic outcomes, the term 'proof' is generally reserved for mathematical, not scientific, conclusions. Research is specifically aimed at generating support (rather than proof) for hypotheses, and, because of the nature of hypothesis testing, a lack of support for the research hypothesis does not refute or provide evidence against the hypothesis. This explains the bias

[1] Don't confuse Type I and Type II errors with statistical error which represents an estimate of sampling or measurement of error within the study.

in the literature toward reporting significant outcomes rather than non-significant ones. It is far more difficult to conclude that certain factors are not related to the outcome variable than to identify factors that are related to it. In accepting the null hypothesis, the investigator merely attributes variation in the outcome variable to chance—indicating that he/she is unable to detect any effect. But there is no indication as to whether this conclusion might have resulted from a poorly designed study that failed to account for or control the level of random variation (noise) in the study. Only when the investigator provides strong evidence that conditions for detecting an effect were optimal (meaning a high level of 'power' within the study) will a statement regarding a lack of relationship between two variables be given any credibility. More typically, hypotheses, and the theories from which they are drawn, die from lack of support or from competing hypotheses that are better supported.

The above probability for making errors, coupled with the fact that investigators can never fully assume that variation in the outcome variable is attributable to only the independent variables measured in his/her study (versus those that are not measured or controlled) means some degree of uncertainty regarding a research conclusion always exists. Investigators are generally aware of this limitation, qualifying their findings with the well-worn cliché that 'more research is needed'. Indeed, this post-positivist approach recognizes the critical need for multiple studies in the process of theory development and hypothesis testing.

Randomizing Steps

Professor Carolyn Schwartz, University of Massachusetts, Department of Family Medicine and Community Health, Worcester, MA 01655, USA

I think that the most important piece of advice I would give is to create a series of steps which potential participants must do in order to be randomized. These steps might involve an intake interview and completing the baseline questionnaire packet in a timely manner prior to being randomized. This approach ensures that the participant is aware of the commitment and work involved in being in the trial, and makes it more feasible for the investigator to maintain a publishable response rate. The written informed consent would, of course, be done at the intake interview.

Critical questions summarized

Investigators should consider the following questions as they design the hypothesis testing strategy:

- which extraneous and confounding variables need to be measured or controlled?
- which procedures need to be used to measure or control extraneous variables?

Minimizing errors regarding hypotheses

Even though not stated explicitly, much of the planning for a research project is actually designed to avoid confounding and minimize Type I and Type II errors—an important **fourth** step in the research planning process. We have already discussed the need to control for and/or measure extraneous variables. This procedure does more than merely protect against confounding within the study. Controlling extraneous variables experimentally or by sampling specific subpopulations can reduce the amount of unexplained variance in the study (the term in the denominator), and measuring an extraneous variable enables the investigator to move variance from the denominator (unexplained) to the numerator (explained). In the words of Cohen [2], "anything that reduces the variability of observations by the exclusion of sources of variability serves to increase power". And as discussed below, power is one way of ensuring a low level of β within the study.

It is important for the investigator to be aware of the typical strategies designed to ensure low levels of α and β. Some of these may be critical in determining which projects the investigator might consider undertaking and which he/she might forego. For example, in some instances the investigator may not have sufficient resources at hand to carry out a study in a manner that ensures reasonably low error rates.

Lowering Type I error rates by changing the significance level

The probability of a Type I error, or α, is usually set at 0.05 or 5%. As mentioned earlier, α can be reduced by using a more stringent significance level such as 0.01 or 0.001. Although it makes sense to report statistical outcomes that reach significance at the 0.01 or 0.001 level, as this indicates a very low α within the study, there is a consequence in actually moving the threshold criterion from 0.05 to 0.01. Doing so makes it five times more difficult to reject the null hypothesis or, conversely, to accept the research hypothesis and thus declare an outcome as significant. Assuming for the moment that the research hypothesis is actually true, that is the phenomenon truly exists in the population, changing α to 0.01 makes it all the more difficult to accept it as true. Thus, the probability that the investigator might ignore a real effect of the independent variable (or make a Type II error) increases five-fold.

Keeping Type II error rates low: the concept of power

Ensuring sufficient power within the study is critically important for maximizing the conditions for hypothesis testing. Power refers to the probability of rejecting the null hypothesis, and ultimately concluding that a relationship between independent and outcome variables exists in the population.

Power is defined as 1 minus β ($1 - \beta$) indicating that, as β decreases, power increases. Although, as with α, there is no specific level of β that is required in a study, Cohen suggests 0.20 as a reasonable target, resulting in a power value of 0.80 (i.e. 1 minus 0.20) [2]. Using $\beta = 0.20$ and $\alpha = 0.05$, it can be seen that the error rate for making a Type II error (under-interpreting the data) is four times that of making a Type I error (over-interpreting the data). So typically there is a 4 to 1 bias towards making a Type II error over a Type I error.

How does the investigator achieve power of 0.80 (or $\beta = 0.20$)? Within a research study, power is related to a multitude of factors, some of which have already been mentioned. These factors are invariably related to the relative amounts of explained and unexplained variance in the study, as well as to the assumptions that can be made about the distribution of those variances. Specifically, in the ratio of explained to unexplained variance, the higher the explained variance and the lower the unexplained variance, the higher the power. Some procedures already discussed that affect power include:

- the level of measurement of the outcome variable, with higher levels (e.g. ratio data) typically providing greater sensitivity and more predictable structure within the data. Not surprisingly, statistical procedures that can assume such predictable structures can increase power

- use of control procedures and sampling techniques that reduce unexplained variance (measurement or sampling error) in the outcome variable add to the power of the analysis as well

Power as a function of α, sample reliability and effect size

As indicated earlier in this chapter, a more stringent significance level (e.g. 0.01 versus 0.05) decreases α while simultaneously increasing β. The conventional strategy is to set α at an acceptably low level such as 0.05 and then identify and set other parameters to approximate the target β of 0.20. Two factors (beyond those mentioned above) that affect the ratio of explained to unexplained variance, and thus β, are the sample reliability and the effect size of the independent variable. Sample reliability helps keep unexplained variance low within the study, while effect size helps increase explained variance.

Sample reliability refers to the degree to which the sample approximates to the population and this parameter can be statistically represented by the standard error of the mean. The standard error provides an estimate of the precision of the sample and its value is always dependent on the size of the sample[2]. Specifically, the larger the sample size, the smaller the standard error, and, consequently, the greater the reliability or precision of the sample due to a reduction in measurement error

---

[2] The standard error is used to establish confidence intervals around the sample mean. In doing so, the investigator can determine a 95% or 99% confidence interval, that is, the investigator can be 95% or 99% confident that the population mean lies within the interval surrounding the sample mean.

(unexplained variation). Thus, a direct and positive relationship exists between sample size and power.

The issue of sample size is pertinent to the clinical investigator because access to patients or other participants may be the limiting factor of the study. How large does a sample need to be in order to achieve a power level of 0.80? This depends on the anticipated effect size of the independent variable (explained variation), as well as other factors that may reduce unexplained variation. Consider an illustration based on Cohen's power tables [2]. Assuming a fairly strong effect size for the independent variable, as might occur in a pharmacological study that investigates a physiological or behavioral outcome, the investigator would require about 20–25 participants per group to maintain a power level of 0.70–0.80. In contrast, an investigator anticipating only a moderate effect, as might occur when a drug can be tested only at a low dose because of its adverse effects or when the study incorporates more 'social' variables, must consider a sample size of 60–70 participants. The difference between 25 and 65 participants can be costly, both economically and in terms of the investigator's time. Anticipating still weaker effects necessitates increasingly large samples to maintain a power level of 0.80.

Apparent from the foregoing discussion is that, in order to achieve a power level of 0.80, there is a trade-off between sample size and effect size. As sample size gets larger, the effect size required for achieving a power level of 0.80 gets smaller, and vice versa.

Effect size refers to the degree to which the independent variable is actually related to the outcome variable in the population. If the effect size is zero, indicating no relationship between independent and outcome variables, then the null hypothesis is true. If the effect size is greater than zero, then the research hypothesis is true. Of course, the research hypothesis will be accepted by the investigator as being true only when the effect size (explained variance) stands out clearly against the background of noise (unexplained variance). As a result, the greater the effect size, the greater the explained variance relative to the unexplained variance, and the more likely the investigator will be able to detect the effect and thus accept the research hypothesis.

Conceptually, effect sizes range from small to large, with their statistical representation depending on the type of research design and analysis being employed. A large effect might be viewed as a difference in standard deviation of 0.80–1.00 between groups or conditions, by an r-value from a correlational study of 0.50, or by an R^2 value in a multiple regression study of 0.25. Whatever the case, understanding and anticipating an effect size for independent variables is useful in determining the practicality of designing and carrying out a study. For example, if the investigator knows that the effect is likely to be small, he/she will either have to expect to use a large sample or look for other ways to reduce unexplained variance through control procedures, sampling techniques, and so on.

Some Examples of Effect Size [2]

	t-test (d)	ANOVA (f)	Pearson (r)	Regression (R^2)
Small	0.20	0.10	0.10	0.02
Medium	0.50	0.25	0.30	0.13
Large	0.80	0.40	0.50	0.26

d: the difference of the means divided by the population standard deviation, or alternatively, the z score difference between the means
f: the standard deviation of the means divided by the population standard deviation
ANOVA: analysis of variance

Critical questions summarized

Investigators should address the following questions as they consider the interpretability of their results:

- what are the acceptable levels of α and β?
- what effect size is anticipated by the independent variable?

- what sample size will be required to achieve a high level of power?

- what other strategies might be used to keep β low?

Simple or complex research designs?

In their enthusiasm to answer too many questions at once, there is a tendency among novice investigators to design studies that are overly complex. Investigators often fail to recognize that even projects that are initially very simple may quickly become complex for reasons beyond the investigator's immediate control.

Reasons to keep the design simple

Simple research designs, having only a few outcome and independent variables, have several advantages:

- the more variables under investigation, the more complex the design must become in order to handle extraneous variation from order effects (does drug before placebo have the same effect as placebo before drug?)

- the number of participants required for simple designs is always fewer—each added variable will necessitate an increase in the sample size in order to maintain a constant power level. For example, in statistical analyses that compare across cells, each new independent variable may cut the cell size in half. In multiple regression analysis, an increase of 5–10 participants may be necessary with each added independent variable

- related to the preceding point, a study with only one independent variable tests for a single main effect, whereas one with three independent variables will test for three main effects and four potential interaction effects among the independent variables. Each new effect, whether main or interaction, uses up a 'degree of freedom' in the analysis, thereby making it more difficult to achieve a significant effect for any one variable

• simple designs often enable the investigator to draw conclusions with fewer qualifications

Why study designs become complex

The advantages of simple designs must be balanced with the potential need for (and benefit of) more complex designs. In the process of designing a study, potential confounding variables may require statistical control. For example, in the cardiovascular study, patients may be drawn from four or five different clinics, meaning the clinic site may contribute extraneous variation (measurement error) and thus must be treated as a 'nested' variable in the analysis. Other factors relevant to the outcome variable may need to be assessed such as: cardiovascular health at pre-testing, age and sex of the participant, family history of disease or daily exercise regimens. By collecting information on each of these, the investigator may be able to move variance from the unexplained to the explained variance category. However, in doing so, each new variable adds to the complexity of the study design, and to all the disadvantages inherent in those designs.

A second clear benefit of complexity is that it allows the researcher to investigate clusters of independent variables both in relation to the outcome variable and to one another. Such designs are often better at simulating real-life situations and

Learning As You Go Along

Dr David Rowland, Professor of Psychology, Dean of the Graduate School, Valparaiso University, Valparaiso, IN 46383, USA

As an investigator of sexual response, I sometimes show subjects stimuli that are erotic in nature. Such stimuli are often interspersed with neutral (non-erotic) stimuli so sexual response returns to baseline between erotic episodes. Imagine my surprise and chagrin when I found that occasionally subjects became sexually aroused to our non-erotic stimuli consisting of clips from the Muppet Show. This of course invalidated the results for these subjects and led to changes in the protocol. But my lesson was that subjects' responses are often completely unexpected and therefore it is important, if possible, to scan each subject's data immediately upon collecting it. This enables the investigator to learn from the protocol as the experiment progresses rather than when it may be too late. As a footnote, in querying subjects about their arousal response to the Muppets, one indicated that Miss Piggy had a slight resemblance to one of the characters in the erotic videotape. Oh well...!

permit the estimation of the relative effect of each variable on the outcome in the context of other potentially relevant variables. For example, the investigator could assess the relative effects of both diet and exercise on cardiovascular health, determining which might be more salient. He/she could also include the age of the participant as an interaction term to assess whether either of these variables has differential effects that are age-based. In conclusion, complex designs enable the investigator to answer a basic research question regarding cardiovascular health in a sophisticated and detailed way that is not allowed by simple designs.

Consider a pilot study first

Sometimes a proposed study becomes unwieldy with variables so quickly that it is wise—as a **fifth** step—to consider running a pilot study before investing significant resources in the project. Pilot studies are, by definition, fairly simple in design and allow the investigator not only to test the protocol but also to get a handle on the effect size of the independent variables. If, after running a handful of subjects, the relationship between the independent variable and outcome variable begins to emerge, the investigator might assume a fairly large effect size and proceed with a more adequate and complex test of the hypothesis.

Not all research is aimed at hypothesis testing, some is aimed at estimation

As stated above, the fundamental statistical tool of the clinical investigator is hypothesis testing, which is used to determine whether the evidence provided by the sample is sufficient to reject the null hypothesis in favor of the research hypothesis. Although most clinical research utilizes this approach, a primary or secondary goal of many studies is to estimate characteristics of the population from the sample under study. Specifically, while rejecting the null hypothesis can lead the investigator to the conclusion that an independent variable has a real effect on an outcome variable in the population of interest, the test itself does not inform him/her about the size or magnitude of this effect. Estimation procedures, on the other hand, offer clinical investigators a means of obtaining an estimate of the magnitude of the effect of an independent variable in the broader population, as well as a measure of the degree of precision of this estimate. Such estimations of the population are achieved by using the 'partial' information provided by the sample, which represents a subset of the population.

The logic behind estimation

The following simple example illustrates the logic behind this estimation process. Suppose that a investigator is interested in some measure of average cardiovascular health outcome for a population of individuals. To estimate this particular characteristic of the population (μ), called a parameter, the mean health outcome for a sample of individuals ($\bar{x}$), called a statistic, can be used as an estimator. The statistic calculated from the partial information provided by the sample is unlikely to estimate the population parameter exactly and any difference between the two is called sampling error. The question then arises about the accuracy of this estimate. To provide a measure of the precision of the estimate, a confidence interval is constructed. A confidence interval represents the range of values around the sample mean that presumably contains the true value of the population mean. This interval is expressed with a predetermined degree of confidence indicated as a probability (e.g. 95% or 99%).

From a conceptual standpoint, a confidence interval is constructed from information about how the estimates of the population (derived from the sample statistic) vary from sample to sample. The commonly used 95% confidence interval produces an interval around the sample mean that contains the true value of the population mean in 95 of every 100 samples. As such, the investigator can be 95% confident that the interval constructed for a given sample includes the true mean of the population, and more specifically in this case, the true mean cardiovascular health outcome.

The size of a confidence interval is, as indicated previously in this chapter, the best measure available to estimate the reliability or precision of the sample: for a given degree (probability) of confidence, the smaller the interval the more accurate the estimate. For many estimators, confidence intervals take the general form 'value of statistic ± margin of error'. For example, if a survey estimates that 55% of physicians favor prescribing generic over brand name drugs, with a margin of error plus or minus 3%, we can be 95% certain that between 52% and 58% of all physicians in the population favor generics, or alternatively, that the error in the estimate of 55% is no more than 3%.

Estimation versus hypothesis testing

The inferential tools of hypothesis testing and interval estimation are used to address different questions. Hypothesis testing is designed to assist the investigator in making a decision about the credibility of a research hypothesis. Estimation is designed to assist the investigator in quantifying the relationship defined by a research hypothesis, without necessarily assuming its credibility. Interval estimation and hypothesis testing are related. As mentioned previously, smaller confidence intervals reflect greater sample reliability, a factor that has direct bearing on power and the consequent likelihood of making a Type II error. Furthermore, a confidence interval can even be used to determine statistical significance. For instance, in the above example, the null hypothesis that 50% of physicians favor generic drugs (the percentage expected by chance) is rejected at the 5% level of significance since this hypothesized value does not reside in the 95% confidence interval with endpoints 52% and 58%. Confidence intervals are very informative because they are probabilistic statements of what is known about the magnitude of an effect.

Choosing statistical analyses

The heart of clinical research entails drawing conclusions about a population of subjects from evidence provided by a sample (subset) of those subjects. The research process itself involves stating a hypothesis that specifies the relationship between two or more well-defined variables, generating a sample of data and selecting appropriate statistical procedures for drawing conclusions from these data. The conclusions rely heavily on the statistical tools of hypothesis testing and estimation. While the basic logic of hypothesis testing and estimation explained above is the same for any clinical research study, a wide variety of statistical techniques are used to implement this logic, depending upon the nature of the research questions addressed and the type of data used. Good estimates and valid hypothesis tests require choosing appropriate statistical procedures—an important **sixth** step in understanding and preparing for the research process. In the broadest terms, statistics can be used to:

- describe the characteristics of the sample

- estimate population parameters from the sample

- describe the relationship between two or more variables using measures of relatedness or association (these procedures often produce an estimate of effect size)

- test the null hypothesis by determining the significance of an outcome

Some or all of the above uses of statistics may come into play in any given project. The latter two rely on the concepts of explained and unexplained variances and typically involve some sort of hypothesis testing at some point in the process. But the goals of the study, the nature of the data, the process by which the data were generated and the presumed nature of the relationship between the variables are all important factors in determining the exact statistical procedures that are to be employed.

I'm not a statistician, what do I really need to know about statistics?
A wide variety of statistical analyses are used in clinical research, some of which are quite sophisticated. In choosing the

appropriate statistical analysis and interpreting the results, a clinical researcher is not expected to fully understand the range of available statistical techniques and procedures. What is important is that the investigator has a thorough understanding of the data, how they were generated, a working knowledge of statistical reasoning, a familiarity with commonly used statistical procedures, the ability to recognize potential pitfalls, and a willingness to include a statistician among the collaborators in the research study if the need should arise. Collaboration between the investigator and a statistician when choosing the appropriate statistical analysis and interpreting the results can be critical to the success of the study and is becoming increasingly common in clinical research. The possible need for inclusion of a statistician should be addressed, especially by the novice clinical investigator, long before the study has actually begun. Obtaining statistical expertise may represent a significant cost to the project, although within some circles this expertise may be bartered in exchange for co-authorship.

First, know your data by generating descriptive statistics

Regardless of the design or type of study, before beginning any kind of involved statistical analysis, the investigator should generate basic descriptive statistics on all the measures of interest. This may include frequency distributions and measures of centrality (e.g. mean or median) and dispersion (e.g. range or standard deviation) for independent and outcome variables, both overall and for subsets of groups or conditions. A careful review of these values can provide the investigator with a sense of whether problems might exist in the data set, whether overall expected patterns are evident, and which, if any, relationships show promise for careful exploration and confirmation.

Know the process that generated the data

The appropriate analytical methods to use and the interpretation of the statistical analysis largely depend on how the research data are generated, i.e. where the data come from. The two major types of data used in clinical research studies are experimental data and observational (or correlational) data. Case studies and single subject designs (used sometimes in pilot research or in situations where participants have unusual characteristics or where settings are rare) provide another strategy for clinical research. However, because they are less commonly used in major clinical studies, they are not discussed in this chapter.

In general, the outcome variable in a clinical study depends upon one or more independent variables of interest and a host of extraneous variables, which are not of interest but which potentially influence the outcome variable. The goal of the research study is to investigate the effect (or relationship) of the independent variable(s) on the outcome variable controlling for the effects of extraneous variables. For example, in a study of the effects of a low-fat diet on cardiovascular health, variables that measure baseline health status, demographic characteristics and lifestyle factors would be extraneous variables.

Experimental data used in clinical research are frequently generated by a randomized controlled trial designed by the investigator. In the ideal trial, subjects are randomly assigned to treatment and control groups, with neither subject nor investigator being aware of group membership. Random assignment should result in groups that are similar in terms of extraneous variables, with any difference attributable to chance. Therefore, control of extraneous variables is achieved largely through randomization so that any statistically significant difference in the outcome variables between groups provides evidence that the independent variable caused a change in the outcome variable. When the investigator generates data through a randomized control trial and chooses the appropriate statistical methods for estimation and hypothesis testing, interpreting the results is usually straightforward. Typically it involves a simple comparison of means, i.e. the investigator attempts to demonstrate differences among treatment group means (explained variance) that stand out against an estimate of unexplained variance (e.g. the random variance occurring within the groups). To make these comparisons, the investigator should have a working familiarity with statistical procedures like the *t*-test, chi-square test, and analysis of variance (ANOVA). Statistically significant outcomes are usually given a causal interpretation—over the past decade, such 'inferential' statistics have been increasingly supplemented with measures of effect size between independent and outcome variables.

Observational (or correlational) data, on the other hand, are generated by a natural process rather than by random assignment by the investigator. Examples of observational data used in clinical research include cohort, case-control and case-series data. In these situations, the outcome variable is measured for groups of non-randomly allocated subjects who receive different treatments, or a single group that receives a particular treatment. For example, let us assume that the investigator does not randomly assign individuals to either a low-fat or high-fat diet condition, but rather simply identifies individuals falling within these categories, or alternatively simply measures fat intake in a sample of 100 men and women. Because the data on cardiovascular health are not generated by a randomized process, the independent variable(s) of interest (fat intake) is likely to be correlated with one or more extraneous variable(s). Specifically, individuals choosing a low-fat diet may also be inclined to get more exercise, or may possibly have been instructed to do so by a physician for health reasons. Therefore, any observed difference in mean cardiovascular outcome between subjects with low-fat and high-fat diets may be the result of one or more uncontrolled extraneous factor such as exercise or health status that are correlated with diet, not necessarily diet alone. Because of this, observational data are more difficult to analyze and interpret and require the use of relatively sophisticated statistical procedures to control for extraneous variables and other problems that may arise when using non-experimental data.

Observational or correlational data are most often analyzed by a multivariate statistical procedure called regression analysis, which statistically controls extraneous variables so that the separate effect of each independent variable can be estimated and tested. Regression (or correlation) models vary but have a common structure, generally producing statistics that provide measures of relatedness or association (e.g. an r-value, R^2 value or odds ratio). In the popular linear regression model, the outcome variable is a linear function of a set of independent variables, which include both the variable(s) of interest and measurable extraneous variables (together providing measures of explained variance), and an assumed random error term that represents the net effect of omitted factors (unexplained variance). The coefficient attached to an independent variable measures the effect of that variable on the outcome variable, while statistically controlling for the effects of all other independent variables. The methods of estimation and hypothesis testing can then be applied to these coefficients to determine whether the independent variable of interest has a significant effect on (or relationship to) the outcome variable. The results are often given a causal interpretation and in many applications are used to make predictions. However, evidence of causation is compromised by the ever present possibility that strong association between the outcome variable and the independent variable might be attributable to one (or more) important extraneous variable that either could not be measured or was inadvertently omitted from the analysis, and therefore was not statistically controlled. Nonetheless, regression analysis is a powerful statistical tool and when carefully applied can simulate a randomized experiment. When working with non-experimental data the investigator should be acquainted with regression analysis.

Know about other factors affecting the choice of statistical analyses

Whether data are experimental or observational (correlational), the specific choice of statistical test is further driven by several other considerations. In experimental studies, for example, tests for differences among treatment groups are dictated partly by the scale of measurement of the outcome variable. Categorical data may call for a chi-square test, ordinal data for a Mann–Whitney, and interval or higher data for a t-test or ANOVA. All three tests generate statistics that enable evaluation of the null hypothesis. In observational studies, logistic regression assumes a categorical outcome (e.g. did the women become pregnant?) and generates an odds ratio, a measure of association that indicates the likelihood of one outcome (e.g. yes) to another (e.g. no). In contrast, linear regression assumes at least interval-scaled data (e.g. how large was the decrease in blood pressure?) and generates an R^2 value, an overall measure of the proportion of variance in the outcome variable that can be explained by all the independent variables together. Both statistics can be tested for their significance to determine whether the magnitude of the effect should be considered more than a chance event that can then be generalized to the population (i.e. a significant outcome).

Other factors also affect the specific choice of statistical test. For example, the distribution of the outcome variable may be bimodal, truncated at one tail or assume other abnormal shapes. The variance across groups or conditions may not be homogenous, or the variance may change as values of the variable reach certain levels. The relationship between variables may be non-linear or even parabolic. Or the outcome measure may occur partly as a function of time (e.g. failure rate of an artificial heart). Investigators can take comfort in knowing that a statistical procedure has been devised for these and just about every other imaginable situation. Because many such procedures are beyond the understanding of the typical clinical researcher, the inclusion (or at least consultation) of a statistician is an important consideration in the planning of most clinical research projects.

Beware of bias

A major pitfall in statistical analysis is the failure to recognize potential sources of bias or systematic error. The methods of estimation and hypothesis testing can deal only with situations in which sampling error is random. As such, bias of any type can invalidate hypothesis tests, lead to incorrect construction of confidence intervals and therefore threaten the validity of conclusions drawn from research data. Bias can arise from the research design, data generation processes, or inappropriate statistical analyses. It is critically important that both novice and seasoned investigators recognize signs of possible bias.

Bias in experimental studies arises from factors that adversely affect randomization and measurement error. Examples include subjects who refuse to participate if assigned to a particular treatment, those who drop out of the study, or those who don't comply with the treatment regimen. In these cases, measured differences in outcomes between treatment and control groups may result from systematic factors (and thus variance) related to subject choice or errors in measurement, rather than the treatment itself. Important potential sources of bias in observational studies are measurement error, self-selection and bias resulting from omitting relevant variables. For example, in an observational study of the effects of diet on cardiovascular health, the investigator must identify, measure and include in the analysis all important factors related to diet that influence cardiovascular health. Since subjects choose their diet, it is most likely that the type of diet is not determined independently of factors affecting cardiovascular health. Failure to account for any important extraneous factors, observable or unobservable, can result in a biased estimate of the effect of diet and invalidate hypothesis tests.

It is important for the investigator to attempt to minimize bias— a critical **seventh** step in the research process. Before a clinician embarks on a research endeavor, he/she should be fairly confident that most conditions that might produce bias in the data (e.g. self-selection) can be addressed. If not, they may present a serious obstacle to carrying out a credible research project. The above mentioned sources of bias, if unavoidable, can sometimes be mitigated using appropriate statistical techniques. Examples of such techniques include self-selection corrected regression models, fixed effects regression models and instrumental variable estimation procedures. Since these analyses tend to be more difficult to implement and interpret, the investigator is encouraged to consult a statistician for assistance.

Critical questions summarized

As investigators determine their strategy for data analysis, they should ask:

- whether their data are experimental or observational (correlational)

- if bias might have influenced the data

- what the level of measurement of the outcome variable is

- whether other factors such as the distribution of the data, linearity of relationships and unusual variance patterns might affect the data analysis

Drawing conclusions

Assuming careful planning, preparation and implementation of the study, it is hoped that the process of drawing conclusions from statistical results will be a straightforward exercise. When involved statistical procedures have been carried out, the step of transforming statistical numbers into research conclusions may require the assistance of the statistician. If there is any doubt, investigators should always verify with a statistician that their conclusions follow from the statistical results. Assuming they do, the investigator should recognize the value of the study's conclusions while not overstating them—they are, of course, only probabilistic outcomes and are subject to error. At the same time, the investigator should acknowledge the limitations of the study, and in particular, exercise caution regarding statements of causality if the study is correlational or observational in nature.

Clinical versus statistical significance revisited

A major pitfall related to interpretation of statistical analysis is the failure to distinguish between statistical significance and clinical significance or practical importance. A hypothesis test leads to the conclusion of a statistically significant or insignificant effect of an independent variable on an outcome variable in the population of interest. Statistical significance indicates how likely it is that an observed effect might arise from chance variation, and therefore provides information about the strength of evidence for the existence of an effect. It provides no guidance about what magnitude of the effect is clinically significant—the **eighth** step the clinical investigator needs to consider. For example, the finding that a low-fat diet has a statistically significant effect on plasma cholesterol concentrations is of little practical importance if the size of the effect is a mere 4% reduction.

As was previously mentioned in the discussion on power, statistical significance depends strongly on sample size. If the sample size of a research study is made sufficiently large, it will almost always produce a statistically significant effect, even if the magnitude of the effect is too small to be important. Alternatively, a clinical study may produce an estimate of an effect large enough to be clinically important (e.g. a 10% reduction in mortality), but which is not statistically significant because of the relatively small sample used in the study. The investigator must be sure not to confuse the size of a test statistic (e.g. t-statistic, F-statistic), which is directly related to the strength of evidence for an effect, with the size of the effect itself.

The magical mystery of 0.05

In hypothesis testing, convention dictates that outcomes greater than 0.05 lead to acceptance of the null hypothesis. However, a good investigator will not ignore probabilities falling between 0.05 and about 0.10. While investigators should adhere to the 0.05 criterion, there is no need to be rigid about it. One of the problems of rigidly implemented hypothesis testing is that it makes no differentiation between an outcome that is 0.06 and one that is 0.35, both lead to acceptance of the null hypothesis. The former strongly suggests an independent variable effect whereas the latter does not. Sometimes outcomes that fall close to 0.05 are reported as 'marginally' significant and the thoughtful investigator will determine effect sizes for these independent variables to ascertain whether they might represent important variables that can guide future research projects.

When a research project fails

While it goes without saying that no amount of analytical sophistication can compensate for a poorly implemented study (although it can sometimes help), even well-implemented, properly analyzed studies do not always lead to crisp, irrefutable conclusions with effect sizes that are clinically salient. The nature of science is such that not all research hypotheses are supported, not all effect sizes are impressive, not all confounding variables can be anticipated, and not all results will find the light of publication.

This brings us to the final—and **ninth**—step in the research process. Well before the study begins, the investigator should consider a back-up plan if the project is a 'wash'. Are there subordinate hypotheses that might be tested to shed light on the phenomenon? Are there subsets of variables that might be explored? Could additional participants be added to enhance power? Even in the unfortunate (and not so rare) event that the project fails, assuming the investigator has planned and implemented the study well, there are usually many things to be learned about the phenomenon under investigation and the procedures used to study it. Nevertheless, identifying several alternative strategies before carrying out the research will often provide peace of mind that may not otherwise exist if the investigator senses that the project is headed toward failure.

Reviewing the Important Steps

Before undertaking a research project, a number of important issues should be considered, as these may have direct bearing on the costs and resources required for implementing the study.

- identify the research questions

- define the variables and specify how they will be measured

- identify relevant extraneous and confounding variables

- take steps to minimize α and β

- consider a pilot study to test protocols and assess effect size

- seek advice in choosing the appropriate statistical analysis

- ensure that procedures are in place to minimize bias

- define and provide a clinically relevant interpretation

- identify alternative strategies if the project fails

References

1. Rowland D, Cooper S, Schneider M. Defining premature ejaculation for experimental and clinical investigations. Arch Sex Behav 2001;30:235–54.

2. Cohen J. Statistical power analysis for the behavioral sciences. New York: Academic Press, 1977.

CHAPTER 6
Ethics in
clinical research

Charles Weijer

Before a clinical trial can begin, the investigator must ensure that ethical standards are fulfilled and that a research ethics committee (REC) has approved the study. These steps require considerable time investment on the part of the investigator. However, through careful attention to ethical issues from the start of the planning phase of a clinical trial, the investigator can avoid unnecessary delays in study approval. Whether planning a clinical trial or practicing medicine: "an ounce of prevention is worth a pound of cure".

There are several important reasons why research involving human subjects is closely regulated. Differences exist between clinical practice and clinical research. In clinical practice, the physician's sole obligation is to the patient. Although this obligation remains in clinical research, it may come into conflict with other obligations and incentives. For example, in order to answer a scientific question efficiently, sufficient numbers of patients must be enrolled within a reasonable time period. Furthermore, substantial benefits may accrue to the investigator upon the successful completion of a research subject. Detailed ethical standards for the conduct of research involving human subjects have, therefore, been set out in codes, regulations and guidelines.

The World Medical Association's Declaration of Helsinki is perhaps the best known of these documents. It outlines the responsibilities of the physician/investigator in a series of statements of principle:

- clinical research must be conducted under the supervision of a qualified medical practitioner, conform to generally accepted scientific standards and be reviewed by a research ethics committee (article I.1–I.3)

- the freely given and informed consent of the research subject, or his/her legal guardian, to study participation must be obtained (articles I.9 and I.11)

- research participation must be associated with a favorable balance of benefits and risks, and "concern for the interests of the subject must always prevail over the interests of science and society" (article I.5)

---

focus on...

THE DECLARATION OF HELSINKI

AKA:
World Medical Association Declaration of Helsinki: Recommendations Guiding Medical Doctors in Biomedical Research Involving Human Subjects

WHAT IS IT?
The primary aim of the Declaration of Helsinki is to safeguard the rights, safety and well-being of participants in clinical research.

Within the context of clinical research, the Declaration states:

1. In the treatment of the sick person, the physician must be free to use a new diagnostic and therapeutic measure, if in his/her judgment it offers hope of saving life, re-establishing health or alleviating suffering

2. The potential benefits, hazards and discomfort of a new method should be weighed against the advantages of the best current diagnostic and therapeutic methods

3. In any medical study, every patient – including those of a control group, if any – should be assured of the best proven diagnostic and therapeutic method

4. The refusal of the patient to participate in a study must never interfere with the physician/patient relationship

5. If the physician considers it essential not to obtain informed consent, the specific reasons for this proposal should be stated in the experimental protocol for transmission to the independent committee

6. The physician can combine medical research with professional care, the objective being the acquisition of new medical knowledge, only to the extent that medical research is justified by its potential diagnostic or therapeutic value for the patient

- the physician is obligated to preserve the accuracy of the research results

- the study protocol should indicate that these principles have been complied with (article I.12)

Investigators should familiarize themselves intimately with the Declaration of Helsinki and relevant national regulations or guidelines.

RECs are a social oversight mechanism used to ensure that the appropriate regulations and guidelines are followed. The REC is a local committee, composed of physicians, researchers, other allied heath professionals, an ethicist, a lawyer, and one (or more) community representative, that carries out peer review for ethical acceptability. The review of multi-center trials offers an exception to local review – in the UK, such trials are reviewed both by regional and local RECs. The investigator ought to carefully follow REC procedures for protocol submission; multiple copies of both the clinical trial protocol and additional forms need to be submitted to the REC, usually approximately 1 month in advance of the committee's next meeting. The investigator may be asked to attend a portion of the meeting and answer questions about the study. The REC may subsequently:

- approve the study outright

- approve the study conditionally upon the completion of minor changes

- require major changes

- reject the study outright

In its review of the protocol, the REC is looking for a clear, well-justified and scientifically sound description of the study that demonstrates sensitivity to the ethical treatment of human subjects. As discussed in more detail below, the REC asks questions pertaining to the study's validity and value, informed consent procedures, risks and benefits posed to participants,

focus on...
ICH-GCP

AKA:
The International Conference on Harmonization of Technical Requirements for Registration of Pharmaceuticals for Human Use Guideline for Good Clinical Practice

WHAT IS IT?
ICH-GCP represents an attempt to provide a mutually accepted standard for the acceptance of submitted clinical trial data in the US, Europe and Japan. The Guideline sets out procedures that should be followed when generating clinical trial data that are intended to be submitted in these markets.

The purpose is to make recommendations on ways to achieve greater harmonization in the interpretation and application of technical guidelines and requirements for product registration in order to reduce or obviate the need to duplicate the testing carried out during the research and development of new medicines. The objectives of such harmonization are a more economical use of human, animal and material resources, and the elimination of unnecessary delay in the global development and availability of new medicines whilst maintaining safeguards on quality, safety and efficacy, and regulatory obligations to protect public health.

WHO DREW IT UP?
The ICH-GCP guidelines received input from hundreds of good clinical practice (GCP) experts throughout the world—some responsible for the set-up and conduct of trials, others for the auditing, inspection or assessment of trials. Despite at times sounding somewhat legalese, drafting was not performed by lawyers—although obviously legal representatives were involved to ensure that the wording did not contravene existing rules.

WHEN WAS IT DRAWN UP?
1996

procedures for subject selection, need for monitoring study conduct and publication (see Table 6.1). Careful attention to each of these issues in the study protocol will minimize both the need for further questions by the REC and the associated delay. If aspects of the study appear to raise ethical issues, the investigator would be wise to discuss them with the REC chair or an expert in research ethics before the protocol is submitted for review.

Validity and value
The clinical trial must pose a clear question and be appropriately designed so as to be likely to answer it in a convincing manner. Justification for the study must be clearly articulated and a clear overview of both pre-clinical and clinical research ought to be

Table 6.1. Questions considered by the research ethics committee in the review of a clinical trial.

Validity and value
- Is the scientific method to be employed valid?
- Is the planned statistical analysis appropriate, i.e. is it likely to provide valid and unbiased answers to the study question?
- Has the investigator demonstrated that the research has scientific or medical value?

Informed consent procedures
- Does the information given to prospective subjects adequately inform them of what is being studied and why, provide details about study procedures, known risks and benefits, uncertainties about risks and benefits, and alternatives to participation?
- Have subjects been told of their right to withdraw from the research without penalty or loss of benefits to which they are otherwise entitled? Have they been advised of any consequences of withdrawal?
- Will there be any costs associated with participation? If so, have these been disclosed?

Risks and benefits
- Do therapeutic procedures fulfill the requirements of clinical equipoise, i.e. is there genuine uncertainty as to the preferred treatment?
- If there is a placebo control, has its use been justified adequately?
- Have the risks associated with non-therapeutic procedures been minimized?
- Is the importance of the research question sufficient to justify the risks associated with non-therapeutic procedures?

Subject selection
- Have the eligibility criteria been justified? Do they strike a reasonable balance between scientific validity and generalizability, i.e. is the study population sufficiently restricted to yield interpretable results without being unduly restrictive?

Monitoring study conduct
- How are subjects to be recruited? Will they be remunerated? If so, is the amount, or nature, of the remuneration appropriate?
- What quality assurance and audit procedures are to be conducted by the sponsor?
- Are additional monitoring procedures required?

Publication
- Has the sponsor imposed any restrictions on the publication of study results? If so, are these restrictions appropriate?

presented. While review of the scientific content is not the primary task of the REC, the committee must ensure that the design is likely to result in the production of valid results. An invalid study cannot be approved, even if risks to participants are minimal. The study must also ask a question of some importance; a study that asks a trivial question, even if it is designed properly, is unlikely to be approved.

Informed consent procedures

Informed consent refers to the ongoing conversation between the investigator and research subject on research participation. The investigator is required to disclose honestly the purpose and details of the study, as well as answer any questions that the participant may have. The consent form itself serves only as a legal document, providing written proof that consent was obtained. In keeping with this understanding of consent, the investigator ought to ensure that new information is given promptly to study participants and further questions are answered as the study progresses.

In addition, the patient should be informed that participation is voluntary and that he/she is free to withdraw from the trial at any time without negative effects on treatment or the relationship with the investigator.

The investigator must disclose the following information to prospective study participants:

- the purpose of the study
- who is sponsoring the research
- why the subject has been approached for study participation
- procedures administered with therapeutic intent, as well as the risks, benefits and uncertainties associated with these procedures
- procedures performed solely to answer the scientific

question (and not administered with therapeutic intent), as well as the risks and uncertainties associated with these procedures (by definition, there are no benefits to the research subject)

focus on...
INFORMED CONSENT

WHAT IS IT?
Informed consent is central to the Declaration of Helsinki, as part of a commitment to protect the rights, safety and well-being of subjects participating in clinical trials.

The ICH-GCP definition of informed consent is:

"A process by which a subject voluntarily confirms his/her willingness to participate in a particular trial, after having been informed of all aspects of the trial that are relevant to the subject's decision to participate. Informed consent is documented by means of a written, signed and dated informed consent form."

However, in some countries informed consent can be verbal rather than written, and in others obtaining informed consent is not a standard component of the clinical trial process.

HOW DO YOU OBTAIN INFORMED CONSENT?
Obtaining informed consent is one of the principal responsibilities of the investigator. Many of the other responsibilities in a clinical trial can be devolved to colleagues, but obtaining informed consent cannot.

If you're participating in a sponsored trial then the sponsor will probably have provided a template informed consent form. You need to read it and make sure that it is written clearly and that the content is appropriate.

Assuming that you do, then the next step is to secure approval from your local ethics committee for the informed consent form and the procedures that you anticipate going through to obtain informed consent from subjects.

Arguably, it is impossible to ensure that someone is 'fully' informed. However, there are various points that you must get across – irrespective of the trial – the most important being that subjects can withdraw from the study at any time without having to give any reason and without jeopardizing their future treatment.

PRACTICAL TIPS
Arrange a room away from the hurly-burly of your clinic where you can spend uninterrupted time with potential subjects. Make sure that all staff members involved in the trial and who the subject may come across are available to meet the subject— especially if you as investigator won't be 'hands on' for much of the trial.

Invite potential subjects to bring their partner or a friend to the interview. Provide subjects with a written summary and give them 24 hours or so to consider. Make yourself available at a specified time to answer further questions.

An informed patient is more likely to be compliant with the trial regimen, so it's worth making that extra effort in the patient interview.

- a detailed description of alternatives to study participation, including alternative treatments

- whether compensation for research-related injury is available

- research subject rights:

  - the right not to participate – non-participation will not adversely affect the care the subject will receive

  - the right to ask questions

  - the right to withdraw from the study at any time

Investigators ought to explore ways of improving the research subject's understanding of the study. This could be achieved by allowing participants to take the consent form home so that they can discuss its contents with both family and friends. Alternatively, pamphlets or a video could be used to present information in a more accessible way. Furthermore, by asking the subject a series of questions following disclosure of the appropriate information, it would be possible to determine whether they had digested the information provided.

focus on...
INTENTION TO TREAT ANALYSIS

WHAT IS IT?

The essential purpose of a randomized trial is to produce treatment groups that are similar apart from random variation, such that any difference in outcome in the trial can be ascribed either to chance or to the allocated treatment.

Since it is possible that deviation from the allocated treatment may be related to outcome, removal of such subjects from the trial can lead to bias.

The statistical device commonly used to obviate such bias is 'intention to treat'.

The principle of intention to treat asserts that data from all randomized patients should be analyzed in the groups to which they were randomly assigned, regardless of their compliance with entry criteria, regardless of the treatment they actually received and regardless of subsequent withdrawal from treatment or deviation from the protocol.

Since it is possible that non-compliance may be related to the outcome of treatment, intention to treat analysis gives a pragmatic estimate of the benefit that a treatment produces in routine clinical practice.

Consent is not only required from the patient, but also from an ethics committee or institutional review board prior to commencing a protocol. The investigator is responsible for obtaining and retaining these approvals. The ethics committee will require:

- the study protocol
- the case report form (CRF)
- details of the financial agreement between the investigator and the sponsor
- details of the indemnity provided to the study either by the sponsor or the investigator

During the study, ongoing updates of any relevant amendments or modifications to the protocol and any safety events occurring on site or at other sites involved in the study need to be forwarded to the ethics committee.

Risks and benefits

Clinical trials typically involve a variety of study procedures. Consider a study of a new antipsychotic drug for the treatment of schizophrenia: patients will be randomized to receive either the new drug or a standard antipsychotic, blood samples will be drawn to measure serum levels of the drugs and psychometric

---

focus on...
STANDARD OPERATING PROCEDURES

AKA:

SOPs

WHAT ARE THEY?

You're likely to hear a lot about the importance of SOPs in the context of clinical trials. Although they sound like management consultant jargon, really they are attempts to ensure uniformity in the conduct of a clinical trial—and you are almost certainly utilizing your own or your hospital's already.

ICH-GCP requires companies to prepare and implement a set of SOPs. Hence, it is very important that all staff at an investigating site are familiar with these and act in accordance with them. One of the aspects of a trial that an audit or inspection will be concerned with is adherence to SOPs.

tests will be used to measure symptoms. The antipsychotic medication, whether experimental or standard, is administered with the intent, in part, of providing benefit to the subject. These are, therefore, therapeutic procedures. The blood samples and psychometric tests only serve to answer the scientific question and are, therefore, non-therapeutic procedures. The risks and benefits of therapeutic and non-therapeutic procedures are evaluated separately by the REC.

Advancing Medical Care

Dr William J Groh, Assistant Professor of Medicine, Cardiology, Cardiac Electrophysiology, Indiana University, 1111 West 10th Street, KI 316. Indianapolis, IN 46202-4800, USA

Clinical research should not be looked upon as a study or protocol that we enroll patients in to make money but as an important method to advance medical care for that patient and for others. Clinical research should be looked at by physicians as something positive they can do for their community. This requires that the physician understands and participates only in trials that he/she thinks are solving important problems.

Therapeutic procedures must pass the test of clinical equipoise; there must exist a state of genuine uncertainty in the community of expert practitioners as to the preferred treatment. Prior to the trial start, none of the study treatments can be known to be inferior to the other study treatments or treatments available in clinical practice. This standard is a basic reflection of the physician's duty to provide competent care to the patient. The use of placebo controls is receiving increasing scrutiny from RECs. Generally speaking, a placebo control may only be used when there is no standard treatment available or when study enrollment is restricted to patients who have failed to respond to existing standard treatments. Thus, in the aforementioned clinical trial of a new antipsychotic drug, a placebo control would be unacceptable because effective treatments for schizophrenia are available. A placebo control would only be permissible in the evaluation of the new drug in patients who failed to respond to standard treatment and for whom no proven second-line treatment exists.

Non-therapeutic procedures do not offer subjects the prospect of benefit and, accordingly, a risk-benefit calculus is inappropriate. In these cases, two conditions must be fulfilled:

- the risks associated with such procedures must be minimized, if possible by obtaining the information in another way, such as by 'piggy-backing' tests on routine medical interventions

- the risks posed by such procedures must be deemed proportionate to the knowledge that may reasonably be expected to be gained from the study. Thus, the ethical analysis of non-therapeutic procedures actually involves a risk-knowledge calculus

Subject selection

Research subjects must be selected equitably; research must neither exploit the vulnerable nor exclude those who may benefit from study participation. Each criterion for study eligibility ought to be justified in the protocol. If the study involves healthy volunteers, it may be permissible to pay subjects for study participation. However, remuneration ought to be carefully justified to the REC. It is unproblematic to reimburse research subjects for any expenses incurred, such as the cost of taxis or a babysitter. Payments to healthy subjects are typically proportionate to the hourly wage paid to an unskilled laborer. An additional sum may be added to compensate for arduous study procedures, if any.

Monitoring study conduct

The REC has a responsibility to ensure that the study will be conducted as approved. Typically, the investigator must provide the REC with an annual update of the number of subjects recruited, and information on outcome and toxicity. When a clinical trial is conducted on a vulnerable patient population, such as persons with dementia, additional procedures may be imposed to ensure that subjects are capable of providing

focus on...
AUDITS AND INSPECTIONS

WHAT ARE THEY?

Ensuring appropriate quality of work in clinical research is essential, both for the protection of subjects involved in the research and also to ensure that the data generated are suitable for subsequent analysis.

There are various mechanisms that operate to ensure appropriate quality. First and foremost there is the protocol. The protocol has to be approved both internally, by a board within the pharmaceutical company (for a sponsored trial), and externally, by the local ethics committee/institutional review board to ensure that the objectives, design and methodology are appropriate.

Subsequently, the investigator and staff at the investigating site should conduct the trial according to the standards laid down by ICH-GCP and approved SOPs.

During the trial, each investigating site will be working with a clinical trials monitor from the sponsoring company. In addition to facilitating communication between the sponsor and the site, the monitor will be on the look out for aspects of trial conduct that need to be improved and will be working with the site to effect any necessary changes.

The official mechanism for ensuring quality is the clinical audit. A clinical audit is a systematic and independent examination of trial-related activities and documents conducted by an independent quality assurance unit within the sponsoring company. Audits are also conducted by regulatory authorities and such cases are termed 'inspections'.

WHY AUDIT?

Pharmaceutical companies are legally accountable for the conduct of the clinical trials that they are running. Audits and inspections are designed to determine whether a trial is being conducted according to the protocol, SOPs, ICH-GCP and any locally applicable regulatory requirements. In the event that problems are uncovered, a variety of sanctions are available to the auditor, against both the sponsor and the investigator.

WHEN DO AUDITS OCCUR?

Audits can be what is termed 'for cause' – i.e. where problems have been identified or are suspected – or part of a random screening process. They can take place both during and after the study. You will usually receive advance notification of an audit. In such a case, ensure that you warn all personnel who will need to be available for questioning during the audit.

SHOULD I BE WORRIED?

If you have been conducting the trial appropriately and have kept all documentation up to date then you should have nothing to fear from an audit. However, it is a sad fact that audits and inspections frequently uncover problems.

Common reasons include:

- inadequate or missing source documents, or source documents that contradict information on the case report form
- protocol non-adherence
- problems with informed consent—either missing, not filed or not obtained
- problems in investigational product handling
- ethics committee approval missing or not complied with

consent and that this consent is properly obtained. Investigators ought to inform the REC of quality assurance and audit procedures that will be implemented by the sponsor.

Publication

The participation of subjects in a clinical trial achieves nothing unless the results are made available to the clinical community. Accordingly, researchers ought to assure the REC that they intend to seek publication of study results upon the completion of the clinical trial. The sponsor has a legitimate interest in protecting proprietary information. It is reasonable for the sponsor to require a 30–60 day publication delay so patents may be sought. The sponsor may not insist upon longer delays, nor may it prevent the investigator from informing research subjects or clinicians of any untoward effects associated with study treatments.

Important ethical documents
International

Council for International Organizations of Medical Sciences. International Guidelines for Biomedical Research Involving Human Subjects. Geneva: CIOMS, 1993.

Nuremberg Code. In: Reich WT, editor. Encyclopedia of Bioethics. Rev. ed. New York: Simon & Schuster MacMillan, 1995:2763–4.

World Medical Association. Declaration of Helsinki. Rev. ed. 1996.

National

Medical Research Council of Canada, Natural Sciences and Engineering Research Council of Canada, Social Sciences and Humanities Research Council of Canada. Tri-Council Policy Statement: Ethical Conduct for Research Involving Humans. Ottawa: Public Works and Government Services Canada, 1998.

Royal College of Physicians. Guidelines on the Practice of Ethics Committees in Medical Research Involving Human Subjects. London: Royal College of Physicians of London, 1996.

United States Department of Health and Human Services. Protection of Human Subjects 45. Code of Federal Regulations 46.

Further reading

Dickert N, Grady C. What's the price of a research subject? Approaches to payment for research participation. N Engl J Med 1999;341:198–203.

Freedman B. Equipoise and the ethics of clinical research. N Engl J Med 1987;317:141–5.

Freedman B, Fuks A, Weijer C. Demarcating research and treatment: A systematic approach for the analysis of the ethics of clinical research. Clin Res 1992;40:653–60.

Levine RJ. Ethics and Regulation of Clinical Research. New Haven: Yale University Press, 1988.

National Commission for the Protection of Human Subjects of Biomedical and Behavioral Research. The Belmont Report: Ethical principles and guidelines for the protection of human subjects research. OPRR Reports 1979(Apr 18):1–8.

Office for the Protection from Research Risks. Protecting Human Research Subjects: Institutional Review Board Guidebook. Washington DC: US Government Printing Office, 1993.

Silva MC, Sorrell JM. Enhancing comprehension of information for informed consent: A review of empirical research. IRB: A Review of Human Subjects Research, 1988;10:1–5.

Smith T. Ethics in Medical Research: A Handbook of Good Practice. New York: Cambridge University Press, 1999.

Weijer C. Placebo-controlled trials in schizophrenia: Are they ethical? Are they necessary? Schizophr Res 1999;35:211–8.

Weijer C, Dickens B, Meslin EM. Bioethics for clinicians: 10. Research ethics. Can Med Assoc J 1997;156:1153–7.

Weijer C, Shapiro S, Fuks A et al. Monitoring clinical research: An obligation unfulfilled. Can Med Assoc J 1995;152:1973–80.

CHAPTER 7
Integrity in clinical research

Philippa Easterbrook

There is no means of knowing how much scientific research is inaccurate or fraudulent. While dishonest or unfair practices are not completely absent from research, in general they are rare. Yet, the findings of one survey in the US which stated that 36% of doctoral and postdoctoral students were aware of instances of scientific misconduct and that 15% were willing to do whatever was necessary to get a grant or publish a paper is of concern [1]. A further study identified considerable disparity among and between scientists and research administrators as to what constituted unethical behavior and how it should be dealt with. For example, 90% of administrators thought that failure to acknowledge an idea that originated in casual conversation definitely should be punished, whereas only 67.2% of the researchers thought so [2]. These findings suggest that there is a need for standards of research integrity and a protocol for consistent actions when misconduct is identified. Ultimately, integrity in scientific research is dependent on individual conscience and commitment. Without the basic assumption that another person's word can be relied upon, the whole scientific research enterprise would quickly unravel. However, it is important that those undertaking clinical research receive practical guidance on the types of unacceptable behavior that may occur, expectations as to reasonable behavior and what to do if things go wrong.

Research misconduct

The Commission of Research Integrity established by the US Department of Health and Human Services together with Congress has defined research misconduct as "significant behavior that improperly appropriates the intellectual property or contributions of others; that intentionally impedes the progress of research; or that risks corrupting the scientific record or compromising the integrity of scientific practices. Such behaviors are unethical and unacceptable in proposing, conducting or reporting research, or in reviewing the proposals or research reports of others" [3]. A few of the more widely recognized examples of research misconduct are discussed below, although it should be noted that the previously accepted definition of research misconduct as 'fabrication, falsification and plagiarism' has now been replaced by three broader categories: 'misappropriation, interference and misrepresentation'.

Plagiarism

Plagiarism is defined as presenting the documented words or ideas of another as your own, without appropriate attribution. The spectrum of plagiarism in research is rather broad, but historically the focus has tended to be on cases of flagrant copying. While block copying of text is a more obvious misdemeanor than appropriating someone's ideas, it is usually less damaging. More sinister practices include the use of information obtained while serving as a grant reviewer or journal referee and the use of a research idea shared with a colleague who does not give you credit for being the source. Often, the individual who has appropriated the idea may claim that they did not realize that this was a definite part of your research activities. When this situation arises, there is often little that can be done, other than to make others aware that they should be careful when sharing their ideas with the individual concerned. The important thing to remember is when exchanging ideas with other researchers, you should be careful to distinguish between the open exchange of ideas that can be followed-up by anyone, the offering of advice, and discussion of your current work and what you are planning to do next. You are also entitled to expect that research data you have collected will be used by you alone, unless you have explicitly agreed to collect the data for someone else or you have specifically given someone else the right to use it, in which case you should receive appropriate credit [4].

Forging

Forging is the invention of some or all of the research data that are reported, including the description of experiments that were never performed. There have been several well-publicized examples of fraudulent research publications in recent years [5–7]. While some were clearly deliberate hoaxes, others appear to have resulted from considerable self-deception. Most of the best known exposures of fraud have been in areas of very active scientific research, where replication of experimental work and critical analysis of earlier work are more likely. However, these and other frauds would have been exposed more quickly if other researchers had maintained a healthy skepticism, and acted on their instincts rather than been so willing to accept the data at face value.

Trimming

Trimming involves the smoothing of irregularities in the data to make the results look more convincing for publication without informing the readers. This temptation to trim may be instilled during school years—a response to the inclination of the teacher to give the highest marks to the student with the smoothest curve!

'Cooking'

Cooking means retaining and analyzing only those results that fit the theory and discarding any inconvenient data. Smoothing experimental data or excluding inconvenient results may seem a minor offence when compared to reporting experiments that were never undertaken. However, the real concern is that the researcher who yields to the temptation in a minor way once and is not found out may well be inclined to do so again, until it becomes a habit.

Misuse of statistical techniques

One area where carelessness, rather than deceit, is a problem is in the misuse of statistical techniques. As in other fields, 'a little learning can be dangerous', and with the ready accessibility of menu-driven statistical packages, many researchers end up using improper techniques without realizing it. For example, in clinical research it is not uncommon for the researcher to rely on computer results without understanding associated hypotheses and assumptions. The computer generates a solution, regardless of the suitability (or not) of the underlying data for a particular statistical analysis. Just as laboratory researchers are expected to know how to prevent contamination of their samples and recognize inadequacies in their equipment, all researchers should have an understanding of the concepts behind the statistical computations and be aware of the limitations of the techniques.

Publication bias

Publication bias is defined as the tendency for authors to submit and journals to publish studies yielding 'positive' results, rather than those with 'null or negative' findings. The existence and extent of publication bias has been widely reported, and the major implication of this is that positive findings of a causal association or benefit of a new drug therapy are disproportionately represented in the medical literature. While the failure to report negative results cannot be strictly regarded as research misconduct, this practice should be discouraged. In addition, researchers undertaking a literature review or meta-analysis (involving quantitative pooling of results) should attempt to access all evidence including unpublished data through a review of, for example, conference abstracts or direct contact with investigators.

Irresponsible authorship

Over the last 10 years, there has been a proliferation in multi-authored papers in the biomedical sciences. While, in principle, it is possible for 20–40 researchers to co-author a single paper, using the term 'author' in the true sense of the word, too often someone is named as an author because of the need to accord recognition rather than because of direct scientific contribution. The spectacle of senior investigators in a multi-center clinical trial jockeying for authorship position to the exclusion of their junior support staff is described hilariously in the poem 'ode to multi-authorship' [8].

Two principles are increasingly being applied to rectify this problem. Firstly, many journals now require manuscript submissions to include a brief section on 'attributions' with the requirement that all persons named as co-authors should have made a major contribution to the work reported. It is certainly unreasonable for your research advisor or head of department to expect their name on every paper published by the laboratory or department as some sort of 'rent' owed to them for making the facilities available. However, it is doubtful whether this approach will resolve the problems of irresponsible authorship.

Secondly, all authors of a paper should be prepared to take responsibility for its contents. Most journals now require all authors to provide a signed assurance that they have read the manuscript prior to submission. Each author must be fully aware of the contents of the paper and declare that, to the best of their knowledge, no substantial portion of the research has been published or is being submitted for publication elsewhere. However, this then raises the issue of how much responsibility authors can assume for the accuracy of the clinical or laboratory data they describe. Responsibilities for the paper are generally limited to each specific contribution from each author. However, by defining each author's role so narrowly and precisely, in effect, it becomes very difficult to hold any of the research team accountable if a problem was identified. In an editorial in the

Ode to Multi-authorship: a Multi-center, Prospective Random Poem

Sir – all cases complete, the study was over
the data were entered, lost once and recovered.
Results were greeted with considerable glee
p value (two-tailed) equaling 0.0493.
The severity of illness, oh what a discovery
was inversely proportional to the chance of recovery.
When the paper's first draft had only begun
the wannabe authors lined up one by one.
To jockey for their eternal positions
(for who would be first, second, and third)
and whom 'et aled' in all further citations.
Each center had seniors, each senior ten bees
the bees had technicians and nurses to please.
The list grew longer and longer each day
as new authors appeared to enter the fray.
Each fought with such fury to stake his or her place
being just a 'participant' would be a disgrace.
For the appendix is piled with hundreds of others
and seen by no one but spouses and mothers.
If to 'publish or perish' is how academics are bred
then to miss the masthead is near to be dead.
As the number of authors continues to grow
they outnumbered the patients by two to one or so.
While PIs faxed memos to company headquarters
the bees and the nurses took care of the orders.
They'd signed up the patients and followed them weekly
heard their complaints and kept casebooks so neatly.
There were seniors from centers that enrolled two or three
who threatened 'foul play' if not on the marquee.
But the juniors and helpers who worked into the night
were simply 'acknowledged' or left off outright.
"Calm down" cried the seniors to the quivering drones
there's a place for you all on the RPU clones.
When the paper was finished and sent for review
six authors didn't know that the study was through.
Oh the work was so hard and the fights oh so bitter
for the glory of publishing and grabbing the glitter.
Imagine the wars when in six months or better
The Editor's response, "please make it a letter".

The order of the authors is not necessarily related to specific contributions, but to the order in which each made their acquaintance with the first author. However, all have made significant contributions to the poem. The authors acknowledge their debt to Theodore Geisel. This letter was originally submitted to the Lancet as an article. RPU= repeating publishable unit; PI= principal investigator. Reproduced with permission from The Lancet, Vol. 348, Number 9043, 1996.

Harold W Horowitz, Nicholas H Fiebach, Stuart M Levitz, Jo Seibel, Edwin H Smail, Edward E Telzak, Gary P Wormser, Robert B Nadelman, Marisa Montecalvo, John Nowakowski, John Raffalli. Departments of Medicine, New York Medical College, Valhalla, New York, NY 10595, USA; Yale University School of Medicine, New Haven, CT; Boston University School of Medicine, Boston, MA; Metrowest Medical Center, Framingham, MA; and Albert Einstein School of Medicine, Bronx, New York.

New England Journal of Medicine in 1983, a case of fraud was discussed where the collaborating clinicians had not been "familiar enough with the techniques to have been aware that their laboratory colleagues had given them a fictitious tracing". Dr Relman concluded: "the lesson seems clear, authors should be familiar with the laboratory tests they write about; otherwise, they risk embarrassing themselves and misinforming their readers…" [9]. If understanding every word or symbol is beyond you, then ideally you should have those sections checked by someone with the appropriate expertise that is not a co-author. Errors can still slip through such checks, but they are more likely to be detected by this responsible approach to authorship.

A distinction between fraud and error

An honest mistake is very different from deliberate fraud, a scientific paper that includes an accidental error may be regarded as just as unreliable. It is not sufficient for the researcher to argue that all research is liable to involve errors. You have a moral obligation to minimize the possibility of error by checking and rechecking the validity of the data and the conclusions drawn.

What should you do if things go wrong?

Science takes pride in being self-policing, but this is a far from straightforward task. Replication of experiments may be flawed and there is often scope for multiple interpretations of data or for clear differences of opinion. Although few researchers in the course of their careers will ever become involved in any of the situations of research misconduct described in this chapter, problems can arise at any time, and it is important to know what procedures should be followed. A first step should probably be to make an initial judgment about the character of the problem. If you come across an apparent error in research findings or techniques by someone else, you should first ask yourself whether this is likely to have been deliberate or accidental. If the error appears to be inadvertent, which will usually be the case, then all that should be necessary is to notify the person concerned directly.

If this approach fails to elicit a reasonable response, further action may be required. An error in a published article, for example, may justify a letter to the editor and be published as an erratum. However, it is important to keep some sense of proportion. A minor error in a paper that is unlikely to have any impact on the message may be unfortunate but does not necessarily require a formal correction or retraction. However, what is to be done if it becomes clear that the error was not accidental or that the conduct of the research was clearly negligent? Again, consider that you may still be wrong in your initial judgment. In such situations, most of us will want to discuss the problem confidentially with someone whom we trust. However, be aware that discussion can easily become gossip, and gossip is a destructive and unscientific way of resolving the situation. If it seems the matter should be pursued, the next stage is to make use of the more formal institutional procedures. Many (but by no means all) institutions have developed guidelines and mechanisms for a proper investigation of the more serious forms of research fraud or negligence. It is essential that anyone who contemplates making use of such a mechanism understands the whole process; what is expected of you and others at each step; and what options there are at different stages of the process to drop the issue.

A few dos and don'ts to help you on your way

- humor is an essential ingredient for successful teamwork. The ability to laugh at yourself and with others is a subtle form of human relationship that alone will prevent internecine disputes as well as being important for maintaining sanity

- be humble in putting forward new ideas by giving credit to those who set you on the right path

- never forget to acknowledge the finance from a grant funding body and those who helped materially (technicians, nurses and secretarial staff)

- never acknowledge help that was not given, even if you think it will please (it will of course, but you may regret it later)

- many who are successful in research become the object of envy and jealousy at some time. Others may belittle your success, cast doubt on your clinical abilities, imply that your work is not important or question your real understanding. Although such remarks are dispiriting, don't brood or let them upset you because the result is inevitably a lower standard of work and a smaller output. Never give into moral blackmail, it is far better to let good work (well-written publications, attention to accuracy, clear lectures) speak for itself

- ethical research behavior depends on group attitudes as well as on individual behavior. If you find that you cannot be part of the solution, do not become part of the problem. Whatever you may have to endure, you should not be tempted to endorse or emulate

Modified from: One way to do research: The A–Z for those who must. Calnan J, editor. London: Heinemann Medical Books, 1976.

References

1   Lock S. Research misconduct. A resume of recent events. In: Lock S, Wells S, editors. Fraud and Misconduct in Medical Research. London: BMJ Publishing Group, 1996.

2   Korenman SG, Berk R, Wenger NS et al. Evaluation of the research norms of scientists and administrators responsible for academic research integrity. JAMA 1998;279:41–7.

3   Commission on Research Integrity. Integrity and Misconduct in Research. Washington: DHHS, 1996.

4   Research as a cooperative activity. In: Honor in Science, Sigma Xi, The Scientific Research Society. New Haven, Connecticut, 1986.

5   Relman AS. Lessons from the Darsee affair. New Engl J Med 1983;308:1415–7.

6   Lock S. Lessons from the Pearce affair: handling scientific fraud. BMJ 1995;310:1547–8.

7   Dyer O. GP struck off for fraud in drug trials. BMJ 1996;312(7034):798.

8   Horowitz HW, Fiebach NH, Levitz SM et al. 'Ode to multi-authorship.' Lancet 1996;348(9043):1746.

9   Relman AS. Responsibilities of authorship: where does the buck stop? New Engl J Med 1984;310:1048–9.

10 Easterbrook PJ, Berlin JA, Gopalan R et al. Publication bias in clinical research. Lancet 1991;337:867–72.

Further reading

Youngner JS. The scientific misconduct process: A scientist's view from the inside. JAMA 1998;279:62–4.

CHAPTER 8
Working with a pharmaceutical company (or other sponsor)
Graeme Moyle

The process of working with a pharmaceutical company should be seen as a symbiosis. All parties involved in the process can gain:

- the company gains through data which may lead to drug approval

- the patient gains through access to new therapies or diagnostics

- the physician gains through the opportunity to work with a new drug, provide this for his/her patients, be given the chance to publish original research and also earn income for his/her research center or hospital

The mutuality of benefit is key to participating in research. Clinical research is highly regulated so physicians should not be, or feel, manipulated by industry and the patient should not be a helpless 'guinea pig' coerced into the process.

The key players involved in the process of development from a new chemical entity to an approved pharmaceutical include:

- the pharmaceutical company developing the compound

- the National Licensing Authority, particularly the Food and Drug Administration (FDA) in the US and the European Medical Evaluation Agency (EMEA) within the European Community

• the investigator

• the volunteers who agree to participate in research trials

Trial designs vary with the development phase and are frequently established by negotiation between the pharmaceutical company development team and the licensing authority, with advice from a panel of expert investigators. In Phases II and IIIa compound safety and activity studies, and any Phase IIIb studies which will be used for regulatory purposes, the relationship between the investigator and the pharmaceutical company differs somewhat from that experienced during Phase IV or post-marketing/post-licensing studies (see Table 8.1). In studies to be used for regulatory purposes, the rigors involved in establishing and conducting a study are substantially greater than in Phase IV studies. More recently, company-led (and much government or research trust run) research has tended to follow similar guidelines. Investigator-led Phase IV studies, not audited or used for regulatory purposes, are generally conducted in a less intensive environment. However, both the FDA and EMEA have issued good clinical practice (GCP) guidance notes for trials of medicinal products, providing principles that should be applied in all research settings.

focus on...
DRUG DEVELOPMENT

Clinical trials are the culmination of an extended period of drug development —which can last for up to 12 years or more from discovery of a lead compound to regulatory submission of data and can cost upwards of $300 million. Given that the patent life of a new compound is only 20 years, this leaves but 8 in which to recoup investment costs. Hence, if a drug makes it into clinical trials, it is essential that these trials are designed and conducted to the highest possible standards.

Key to these issues is the protection of trial subjects, the involvement of an independent ethics committee and the provision of informed consent under the Helsinki agreement. These guidelines also provide information about the responsibilities of the sponsor, the monitor and the investigator,

Table 8.1. Questions considered by the research ethics committee in the review of a clinical trial.

Phase	Subjects	Aim	No. of patients	Duration
Phase I	Healthy volunteers	To determine safety, metabolic effects and tolerable dose levels in humans	20–100	Several months
Phase II	Patients	To determine efficacy against the disease and to identify doses that are both effective and well tolerated	80–400	Several months to 2 years
Phase III	Patients	To confirm efficacy in larger number of patients. May help uncover rare side effects	1000–3000	1–4 years
Phase IV (post-marketing studies)	Patients	To confirm safety in the general population, and physician and patient acceptance of the new medicine. May help uncover rare side effects. May be large scale, long-term studies investigating morbidity and mortality. Phase IV studies often compare a drug with other drugs already in the market, and may also be designed to determine the cost-effectiveness of a drug therapy relative to other traditional and new therapies		

and guidelines on how data should be handled and subsequently archived. Additionally, the financial agreements and issues surrounding ethics and publication are strictly governed in industry sponsored research to avoid influence on investigators and coercion of subjects to participate in a study. Ultimately, these guidelines serve to assure the quality of the information derived from medical research used for drug licensing and approval.

Protection of the trial subject, the Declaration of Helsinki and consent

The process of obtaining the written and informed consent needed for patient participation is performed on the basis of the Declaration of Helsinki. The investigator is responsible for obtaining informed consent before each subject enters any trial and before any procedures related to the trial are undertaken. Under the Declaration of Helsinki, patients should be provided with:

- written and verbal information, in both the local language and layman's terms, describing the trial and providing details of the medication and comparator medication to be used (if any), and explaining any or all alternative treatments available to the subject if they refuse to participate in the trial

- study design (aims, methodologies)

- study procedures

- any potential hazards, risks and discomfort, and the anticipated benefits which may occur through participation

Participation in a clinical trial is confidential; participants are individually identified by initials, date of birth and/or a number to enable source document verification by the sponsor or auditing regulatory authorities without revealing the subject's identity. Additionally, informed consent is an ongoing requirement so the subject should be informed of any relevant new findings in the therapy area and re-consent if any protocol amendments occur during the study. Finally, patients should be given the names and telephone numbers, preferably with a 24-hour availability, of appropriate persons to contact in the case of an emergency.

Indemnity

For drugs in development, the sponsor generally provides compensation through insurance or indemnity. Compensation is provided in the event of injury or death of a subject as a result of his/her participation in a clinical trial. This indemnity additionally insures the investigator against losses resulting from any liability associated with such injuries or deaths.

Arrangements for compensation are conducted according to local laws and, therefore, vary between different countries. In investigator-led research, the investigator or hospital provide their own indemnity insurance.

focus on...

INDEMNITY

WHAT IS IT?

As with any experimental procedure, clinical trials are associated with an element of risk—in this case primarily for the subjects enrolled in the trials.

Indemnity insurance is the cover provided by the sponsor to the investigator in the event of an untoward occurrence resulting in a patient suing the doctor. The cover is not valid in cases of protocol violation and does not cover negligence by the investigator. It is prudent to check the level of cover provided before agreeing to participate in a trial.

Knowing your stuff

Both the sponsor and the investigator are key to the successful running of a clinical trial. The investigator needs to ensure that he/she is familiar with the available data on the product under investigation and maintain his/her knowledge as new information emerges. Generally, this information will, in part, be provided by the industrial sponsor to the investigator as part of an investigational drug brochure. However, once a drug is licensed, this brochure is infrequently updated and, therefore, ongoing medical education by the investigator is essential.

Setting up, curricula vitae and signatures

Research guidelines direct the investigator to provide sufficient time for the conduction and completion of the trial.

The investigator must also provide adequate and appropriately trained staff, appropriate facilities for the patient to attend – which may include dedicated clinic rooms or facilities such as a specific pharmacokinetic unit – and laboratory or sample processing equipment. In agreeing to participate in a study, an investigator should not try to exaggerate the number of patients they may potentially recruit, but provide appropriate

focus on...

THE INVESTIGATOR'S BROCHURE

AKA: IB

WHAT IS IT?

Taking possession of a huge mountain of documentation is an unfortunate corollary of involvement in a trial. Among these documents you will find the IB. The IB is a full account of the clinical and non-clinical data on the investigational product that are relevant to the study of the product in human subjects. Fundamentally, the IB is designed to tell you why the product is being investigated, what investigations have been carried out to date, what has been learnt and its relevance to human subjects, and any special features of the pharmacology, etc. with which you will need to be familiar in order to manage subjects appropriately. In the words of the ICH-GCP:

"The overall aim ... is to provide the investigator with a clear understanding of the possible risks and adverse reactions, and of the specific tests, observations, and precautions that may be needed for a clinical trial. This understanding should be based on the available physical, chemical, pharmaceutical, pharmacological, toxicological and clinical information on the investigational product(s). Guidance should also be provided to the clinical investigator on the recognition and treatment of possible overdose and adverse drug reactions that is based on previous human experience and on the pharmacology of the investigational product."

DRUG DISCOVERY AND DEVELOPMENT

The first and perhaps most important question for a company to ask is "what should we be researching?" Assessing unmet clinical needs – where no suitable therapy exists – is the first step; determining which needs are most significant and which can realistically be met is the next. Researchers then need to identify a suitable target for therapeutic intervention (for example, an enzyme or receptor). On average, 150,000–200,000 compounds are then screened for activity against this target to yield just one lead compound. At this stage, the company has to determine whether development should proceed, and a team derived from departments spanning research through to manufacturing and marketing is responsible for this decision. If the decision is to proceed then a development plan will be put in place, which will carry the compound (assuming that it does not fail earlier) through pre-clinical and clinical testing.

The lead compound may first undergo a series of chemical modifications to optimize its activity and stability. This optimized compound will then advance to pre-clinical testing, primarily to test activity against the target *in vivo* and to gather pharmacokinetic and toxicity data. Assuming that the data warrant such progression, the compound will then move into Phase I clinical testing. Although 150,000–200,000 compounds are screened to yield one lead compound, 80% of these fail to enter clinical testing. Of those that do, only about 10% make it to the market. So for every one new compound to be launched, millions are likely to have been lost by the wayside. The average R&D expenditure of a medium-sized pharmaceutical company is approximately $1 billion.

It's Good to Talk

Dr Neal Uren, Consultant Cardiologist, Department of Cardiology,
Royal Infirmary of Edinburgh, Edinburgh EH3 9YW, UK

Keeping on top of the planning of a new research project is mandatory to ensure that a clinical trial starts on time. I put together an idea, wrote a protocol and took it to a colleague in a pharmaceutical company for funding. He liked the project and showed it to others within the research section, suggesting that it should be funded as a two-center trial. We met up with the company's clinical research team and regularly advised them on the design of the protocol. After several months we identified patients for the study and met up with the company's clinical research organizer who assured us that the study was almost ready to start. Details were passed onto the hospital-appointed body responsible for coordinating research with industry who subsequently conducted their own private negotiation with the company and passed on agreements to the National Health Service (NHS) central legal office. We were unable to find out why the study was being held up, until we discovered that this negotiating body was arguing over the pharmaceutical company's worldwide affiliates and whether they were morally acceptable to the NHS Trust. Basically, the study was delayed because of unnecessary bureaucracy. Two years later, we are almost ready to start and the negotiating body is no longer contracted to the Trust. The moral of the story is that no one has your best interests at heart other than yourself; pharmaceutical companies have their own legal constraints placed on how they negotiate contracts and a middle-man in the Trust adds to the complexity of the situation. To speed things along, you need to maintain regular communication with both the drug company and the Trust's research and development office to ensure that the study is not caught up in unnecessary legal wranglings that will delay onset by some considerable time.

---

patient numbers. This should be based upon database search information, rather than guesswork. However, only experience can guide what proportion of those in the planned trial recruitment period meeting the entry criteria are likely to agree to participate in a clinical research protocol. Each protocol that runs at a center affects the relationship between the investigator and the funding source; failure to live up to recruitment expectations is a common cause of friction between the sponsor and the investigator.

All investigators involved in a study, including both the principal investigator and any conducting investigators at the site, and research staff are required to submit an up-to-date curriculum vitae detailing their credentials and qualifications to the sponsor and, if necessary, to the relevant licensing authority.

focus on...

THE CENTRAL LABORATORY

AKA: The core laboratory

WHAT IS IT?

In multi-center trials it is becoming increasingly common for the sponsor to utilize a single laboratory for analysis of materials. This has the advantage of ensuring standardization of operations. The laboratory may be at one of the sponsor's research sites or it may be contracted in for the duration of the trial. The sponsor will provide appropriate standard operating procedures (SOPs) detailing how samples should be forwarded to the laboratory.

Upon agreeing to participate in a trial with the sponsor, the investigator is required to sign a protocol agreement stating that he/she has read and understood its contents and is willing to work according to the GCP guidelines for medical research. There is usually an agreement with regard to the planned publication policy; publication is generally the combined responsibility of both the sponsor and the investigator. Once the protocol is agreed and signed, submission to the relevant ethics committee is performed jointly with the sponsor. Following ethics committee approval, the investigator should inform both staff members involved in the trial and those involved in the potential trial patient's management about the conduct of the trial. This task is usually performed with the assistance of the sponsor at a study set-up meeting.

Upon recruitment of a participant to a study, the trial subject is required to provide signed informed consent. This should be witnessed by at least two people:

- someone directly involved in the study who has provided the patient with both the written and oral information for consenting into the study

- an independent person to confirm that the consent is informed and that there has been no coercion to enter into the trial

More signatures

At the commencement of a trial, all study personnel involved in recording information in the notes or case report form (CRF) are required to provide a signature page to the sponsor. During the study, results from investigations, as well as any records in the clinical notes, need to be signed by the person entering those records. Upon completion of the study, the investigator will sign the CRF confirming that the data contained within it have been appropriately collected and recorded. The investigator's name is included in the publication and, in general, the accepting journal will require a signature from the investigator confirming that he/she agrees to the submission of the article to the journal.

Handling drugs

Particularly during studies involving investigational medications or products, the sponsor is required by the regulatory authorities to keep a log and record of where that drug has gone. The sponsor provides the investigator (usually the pharmacist) with a drug handling log which will detail both the date and time of delivery from the sponsor to the investigator's pharmacy and subsequently the dispensing of that product to the trial participant. This helps to ensure that investigational products are only dispensed to trial subjects in accordance with the protocol and that unused products are returned to the sponsor. At the end of the study the sponsor and investigator are required to reconcile delivered goods with use and return of stock. Generally, in studies involving investigational medications, study participants are requested to return any unused stock to the investigator or his/her pharmacist at each study attendance.

Unblinding

The investigator and pharmacist are provided with study codes to enable unblinding of a study, in accordance with the protocol, should an adverse event (AE) occur which necessitates full knowledge of the patient's drug regimen. In the instance of such an event, the case should preferably be first discussed with the sponsors and the reasons for unblinding recorded in the participant's notes.

On completion of the study, the sponsor should promptly provide a randomization list enabling the participant's treatment to be recorded in their medical records.

Quality assurance

The key to successful drug investigation is the accurate collection, recording and reporting of data. Information entered into the CRF should also be included in the participant's clinical notes. Events should be recorded either in standard text or accepted shorthand and, in both cases, be recorded in an identical form. For example, if a patient fractured his tibia during a study and 'fractured tibia' was recorded in the notes, 'fractured tibia' should also be written in the CRF rather than 'broken leg'. At the end of the trial, similar AEs will be coded together so that patients who have a 'fractured tibia' and 'broken leg' will be grouped into one AE category. However, for source document verification, it is necessary for events to be recorded in the CRF and patient's notes in the same way. Similarly, all blood, imaging and other investigations need to be included in the notes as well as being provided in the CRF.

Adverse events: serious but not always severe

AEs occurring within a study take two forms: (i) ordinary AEs; and (ii) immediately reportable AEs. Immediately reportable AEs are serious and include:

- a death that occurs either during the trial or within 4 weeks after stopping treatment

- an event which is considered by the investigator to be life-threatening

- an event which may be permanently disabling

- an event which requires in-patient hospitalization of an individual or increases the duration of an in-patient hospitalization

- the development of a malignant neoplasm during the trial

- the occurrence of a congenital anomaly during the trial

- the occurrence of pregnancy during the trial

- an overdose, i.e. a deliberate or inadvertent administration of a treatment at a dose higher than specified in the protocol

These AEs, either clinical or laboratory, may or may not be considered by the investigator to be related to the study medication and must be reported to the sponsor within 1 working day of their occurrence. Importantly, serious AEs are often not severe in intensity (e.g. no one ever has a severe pregnancy). Similarly, events of a severe intensity are not always serious AEs, e.g. 'The injection caused a severe pain which lasted a few seconds but which hasn't recurred.'

Other AEs occurring during the study which do not meet the immediately reportable AE criteria are recorded in the CRF at the next study visit. In general, clinical study protocols provide gradings of severity, (generally grades 1–4, or mild, moderate, severe or potentially life-threatening) and request an investigator's assessment of the event's relationship to the trial or study drug. The most common classifications include unrelated, remotely related, possibly related or probably related. The classification: mild, moderate, and severe or potentially life-threatening, is commonly defined (see Table 8.2). The investigator is responsible for recording the date of the development of the AE and its subsequent follow-up. The outcome of AEs, such as whether the event has stopped or is ongoing, is required. Any treatment required for an AE should also be recorded in the CRF.

focus on...
ADVERSE EVENTS

The distinction between AEs and adverse drug reactions (ADRs) can be a source of confusion. AEs are all undesirable experiences that occur to a subject during the course of a clinical trial—irrespective of any relationship with the investigational drug or device. If the relationship between the product and the event is at least a reasonable possibility then it is considered to be an ADR. Hence, all ADRs are AEs, but not all AEs are ADRs. Events vary in severity. Usually they are classified as either serious or non-serious. A serious AE is one that results in death, is life-threatening, requires in-patient hospitalization or prolongation of existing hospitalization, is a congenital anomaly/ birth defect, results in permanent impairment of function or damage (for medical devices only), jeopardizes the health of the patient or may require subsequent medical or surgical intervention. Others may be included in the trial protocol, and it is the responsibility of the investigator to be aware of these. In a clinical trial, it is the responsibility of the investigator to know the procedures for reporting AEs, including to whom they need to be reported, how they need to be reported and when they need to be reported. The sponsor will have provided a set of SOPs detailing how AEs should be reported within the IB.

WHAT TO DO

All AEs need to be recorded in the CRF and reported, but how do you manage to achieve 'all'? Many such events will occur when the subject is off-site, hence you will need somehow to elicit information from the subjects, without 'leading the witness'. You must emphasize to subjects before the trial starts that they must be frank in reporting potential AEs—however trivial they may appear. Encouraging subjects to keep diaries is a useful tip. Your report should be as comprehensive as possible, so you should include the time, the duration, the severity, any treatment and the outcome. Serious AEs require particular attention and particularly prompt attention too. Investigators should report all serious AEs to the sponsor by telephone immediately (so you need to ensure beforehand that you have all appropriate contact details close to hand) and follow up with a letter. The sponsor may provide a special form for reporting AEs with the CRF. The sponsor is obliged to report all serious AEs to the appropriate regulatory authorities within a short period of time (15 days of receiving the report or 7 days if the event was fatal). You should also report the event to your ethics committee.

DETERMINING CAUSALITY

It is the responsibility of the investigator to assess the causality of each AE. Using clinical judgment, the investigator must assess whether the event is related to the treatment or intervention, may be related or no judgment can be made. Here, clinical judgment is important as the physician will have spent time with the subject whereas the sponsor assessing the report, despite knowing treatment allocation and hence being able to differentiate between AEs and ADRs, will not have.

TREATMENT

Exercise of clinical judgment is essential also in determining whether and what treatment should be provided following (or during) an AE. The IB provides a list of all contraindicated medicines and others whose use will invalidate data analysis and hence necessitate withdrawal of the subject from the study.

Determining appropriate treatment isn't that difficult—after all, the patient will either have been on study drug or control, so you will know what, if any, concomitant drugs or interventions are contraindicated. In some circumstances, however, it may be important to unblind the subject prior to treatment initiation. You need to be aware of the procedures for unblinding and these should be detailed in the IB.

Data provided on serious AEs are then given to the sponsor and subsequently back to the investigator and any relevant authorities, the investigator being responsible for forwarding this information on to the local ethics committee. AEs occurring at other sites involved in the study would also be provided to the investigator by the sponsor and on to the local ethics committee.

Monitoring and auditing

In order to ensure that data are collected and recorded in an appropriate way, clinical trials are generally studied by a monitor, either from the sponsor company or from a clinical research organization employed by the sponsor company. When this person visits the trial site for 'source document verification' (checking the CRF against the clinical record and investigation results), the investigator is required to make notes available. In general, the monitor will pre-warn the investigator as to

Table 8.2. Adverse event classification in a clinical study protocol.

Recorded in CRF	Event criteria
Mild	A discomfort not disrupting normal daily activity
Moderate	A discomfort sufficient to reduce or affect normal daily activity
Severe	An event that leads to inability to work or perform normal daily activities
Potentially life-threatening	An event that is genuinely life-threatening, permanently disabling or leading to hospitalization

which notes are needed. In trials where data may be used for approval purposes, an audit may be performed by an independent audit group from the sponsor company or by a regulatory body such as the FDA or EMEA. In these cases, the investigator is not warned as to which notes will be audited. These visits can be quite stressful but if you have done the job well they can also provide a sense of satisfaction. Additionally, passing an audit forms part of the maturing process as an investigator and is key to building a reputation with the sponsor as a quality research site.

focus on...

THE CLINICAL TRIALS MONITOR

AKA: CTM

Monitoring is an essential part of a clinical trial. The CTM acts as a bridge between the sponsor and the investigator to facilitate the conduct of the trial. Increasingly, CTMs are casting off their 'box checker' image and being used more as 'site managers'—helping to ensure that facilities are prepared before the start of a trial and working with the site to solve problems as they occur.

WHAT IS MONITORING?

The purpose of monitoring is to verify that the rights and well-being of the patients are protected; that reported data are accurate, complete and verifiable from source documents (source document verification); and that the conduct of the trial is in compliance with the protocol, good clinical practice and applicable regulatory requirements. The CTM is responsible for reviewing documents at your site at different stages of the trial. The CTM will visit

your department and review on-site documentation, procedures and other elements involved in the trial. The monitor will require information before, during and after the trial and it is the responsibility of the investigator to make sure that the required information is available. Before the trial you need to ascertain with the monitor the frequency of visits, what the monitor will need to see (i.e. what you need to provide), who needs to be there (e.g. research nurse, pharmacy staff), how long the visit will last and for how much of the time you or members of your staff will be required. It is also very important to establish the means of contacting the monitor (and vice versa) together with alternative contacts should either the monitor or yourself be unavailable.

PRACTICAL TIPS

Value the monitor as a resource. In general CTMs have years of experience in running clinical trials and should be considered an excellent source of practical advice. Utilizing their skills efficiently should make your job as an investigator that much easier. If you can anticipate what might go wrong and head it off then you will be much more efficient—and are more likely to be asked to participate in future trials too.

Patient care

By including a patient in a clinical study, the investigator is responsible for ensuring the confidentiality of information regarding that individual and providing both appropriate medical care and advice during the study. For example, the investigator is required to have fully functional resuscitation equipment available in the event of an emergency during a pharmacokinetic study. If new data emerge during the course of a study that suggests that participation of a particular individual may be detrimental, it is appropriate that the investigator provides suitable medical advice to the patient. Additionally, the investigator is responsible for the follow-up of clinical AEs, as well as any laboratory abnormalities that may be of importance to the subject participating in a clinical trial. Patients in many studies now carry a card, which identifies them as participants in a clinical trial, and also provides a contact address and telephone number if action is needed. Ideally, the contact should be available 24 hours a day throughout the duration of the study.

Following informed consent, it is generally appropriate that the patient's family doctor should also be informed about his/her participation in the clinical study.

focus on...
SOURCE DATA VERIFICATION

WHAT IS IT?

What the trial is seeking to achieve and how it intends to achieve it are described in the clinical protocol. The protocol provides information on the design and methodology; for example, the inclusion and exclusion criteria. A clear, well thought out, well-written protocol is key to a successful clinical trial. Once a protocol has been approved, it is essential that the clinical trial is carried out in accordance with that document. In the context of regular quality assurance checks during a clinical trial, ensuring that data are accurately recorded and transcribed is essential. Source data verification refers to the procedure whereby a CTM directly compares data written in the CRF with that contained within the source documents (e.g. patient files). Often source data verification will be carried out during a study. This is a lengthy procedure and it is therefore important that you arrange for a suitable room for the monitor and that all relevant documentation is available.

The case report form

Through his/her participation in a study, the investigator undertakes to ensure that observations and findings are recorded correctly and completely in the CRF and subsequently signed off. Investigators using computerized systems are required to provide safeguards to ensure that data can be validated. Data print-outs need to be signed and hard copy records kept. Sadly, the days of paperless clinical trials remain a long way off. Depending on the study, the CRF should be signed on every attendance and corrections within the CRF should be initialed. The preferred writing instrument for clinical trials is a black ballpoint pen.

focus on...

THE CASE REPORT FORM

AKA: The case record form or case study form

WHAT IS IT?

In a clinical trial, all data are important. Without a complete picture of what has happened, who it happened to and when it happened, efficient analysis of the trial will be difficult and perhaps compromised. The CRF is the document that contains all the information required by the protocol for a particular patient. A properly designed CRF should ask only for the information that is essential for the subsequent analysis of the trial and be designed in such a way as to facilitate completion by the investigator.

WHO DRAWS UP THE CRF?

In a sponsored trial, the CRF is designed by the sponsoring company. Generally, it is then field tested among a group of investigators and refined to take their comments into consideration. A statistician should be involved in the design phase.

TIPS AND TRICKS

Unfortunately, errors on the CRF are common. Any number of reasons may be responsible, for example time or a user-unfriendly design, but most are avoidable with very simple strategies. Perhaps the most important error is conceptual—think of completing rather than filling in the CRF.

BEFORE YOU START

Don't wait for the first patient visit to run through the CRF. Make sure that you and whoever else will be involved in entering data on the form are familiar with where, when and how data should be entered (including what color pen, etc.). There's no substitute for a run-through of the CRF with the monitor before the start of the trial. You also need to know what to do with the forms once completed.

ENTERING DATA

Before a patient visit, make sure that you have to hand all relevant documentation —including the correct CRF (yes, it happens…), and enter all the required data at the time of the patient visit. (It's unwise to rely on memory and making notes and transferring them runs the risk of letting transcription errors creep in.)

Statistics, analysis and publication

Study protocols detail the primary outcomes for the study. These include a primary endpoint, (generally an assessment of efficacy), additional assessments of efficacy (secondary endpoints) and descriptive analyses of the AEs occurring during the study. Protocols additionally contain details of statistical methods to be employed upon completion of the study for the analysis of the available data. This is generally done to avoid 'fishing expeditions' or 'data mining' if favorable or statistically significant outcomes are not observed over the course of the study. The provision of these statistical methods at the start of the study also enables estimation of the sample size needed.

In setting up a trial, there is generally a discussion between the investigator and the sponsor as to the responsibilities regarding publication. However, this area continues to remain somewhat neglected. Several styles of publication planning exist, although in some cases there is none whatsoever. Often, members of a Steering Committee appointed for the trial may subsequently form the Publication Committee. The authors may then be listed as 'the study group' or in alphabetical order, in which case changing your name to Aaron Aardvark may be helpful. Other studies employ a competitive publication practice; the physician who recruits the largest number of patients into a clinical study becomes the first author on the publication. Publication of other studies is often left to the investigator who is most enthusiastic about contributing to a publication.

focus on...

DATA HANDLING

Clinical trials generate vast quantities of data, and they all need to be recorded, reported and analyzed in an identical manner. Every aspect of data handling, from entry of a measurement on the CRF to publication in a peer-reviewed journal, needs to be conducted in a rigorous manner to ensure that errors and inaccuracy are not allowed to creep in. Too much time and expense are wasted on problems in data handling— unfortunately, most commonly due to problems with completing the CRF.

focus on...
THE STUDY REPORT

AKA: The final report

WHAT HAPPENS TO ALL THE DATA?

You've worked hard completing the CRFs for each of your patients and the CTM has collected them all and taken them away for analysis. What happens next? After checking and statistical analysis, the data are compiled into what is termed the 'study report'. This is a large document that should contain the rationale for the study, the methods (the protocol), the results, interpretation of the results and tabulation and full listings of all the data collected. Whether you as investigator contribute to or review the final report will have been determined in advance. All aspects of data review (including the publication strategy) are determined before the start of the trial. The study report is then submitted to the appropriate regulatory authority—sometimes as support for a product license application; sometimes as additional information. Assuming that there are no (well, no is unrealistic; few may be possible) delays resulting from problems with the data (e.g. errors on the CRF) then the study report will be prepared relatively quickly—a pharmaceutical sponsor has a large number of individuals available to assist. However, if you're writing up your own study then the burden will fall upon your shoulders—if you've written a thesis (or have known colleagues while they were preparing theses) then you know that this isn't a trivial task.

PUBLICATION

As stated above, whether, where and when data will be published or presented will have been determined in advance—as will authorship (who gets to be where on the author list). You should look very carefully at the provisions for publication in the contract provided by the sponsor. Obviously it is desirable that all data are published. However, there are circumstances – usually commercial – in which publication needs to be delayed.

Publication by a committee is rarely successful without one individual taking responsibility. In studies that are key to a pharmaceutical company, provision of a medical writer to the trial Steering Committee is often made. However, care should be taken when dealing with medical writers as they are prone to 'dumb down' information and frequently have limited knowledge of the subject area within which they are dealing. Thus, they may subtract from the quality of the publication, albeit accelerating some parts of the process such as recording the methodology and results. In studies that are investigator-led, it is the responsibility of the investigator to arrange publication, usually by suggesting to a junior doctor that this process will enhance their career or will ensure that they receive funding to attend a glamorous international conference.

Planning and Resourcing

Joseph Pergolizzi, Director of Business Development, John Hopkins University School of Medicine, Department of Internal Medicine, Baltimore, MD 21205, USA

Appropriate pre-emptive staffing for anticipated studies presents many areas of concern. We conducted a Phase III postoperative analgesic study that required four blood samples to be taken after the administration of a single dose of the study drug in the recovery room. This sampling (S1–4) had to be performed 0, 1, 12, and 24 hours post-administration of the study drug, respectively. Pain assessment needed to be performed at the same time as each blood withdrawal. The study was a competitive enrolment study, with an enrolment goal of 20 patients within 3 months. The study budget provided for a principal investigator, one study nurse coordinator and one research assistant. At the investigators' meeting, many sites, including ours, voiced concerns regarding staffing needs for the study. It was felt that the sponsor had not appropriately accessed the amount of time that the team would have to spend with each patient. The sponsor had assumed that each blood sample and assessment would take a maximum of 1–2 hours and had, therefore, based their budget accordingly. Although the actual time allocated per visit may have been correct, we felt that the study budget lacked attention to detail and had not accounted for the actual time that the team needed to be available. If a patient finished surgery at 3 pm for example, the first scheduled study assessment and blood sampling (S1) would be at 3 pm, S2 at 4 pm, S3 at 3 am and S4 at 3 pm the next day. This obviously meant that the coordinating team would have to be present and available throughout the entire time, particularly S3. After we presented our concerns, the sponsor agreed that this would be problematic, especially if there were multiple patients enrolled per day at various times. We all agreed that the provision of two teams would be more appropriate and would assure maximum enrollment within the time lines. The allocation of additional study staff helped us to meet our enrollment goals.

In retrospect, the involvement of a third team would have made it easier to collect the data required, and this provides an example of why we must pay careful attention to the study visit schedule when appropriately coordinating staff efforts. Additionally, the investigators' meeting should always be attended by as many study team members as possible, enabling everyone to become familiar with the protocol and discuss issues with the sponsor before commencing the study. Finally, in-patient clinical studies are usually difficult pain management trials and require experienced study coordinators.

Money

All financial aspects of a trial should preferably be arranged with the study sponsor prior to initiation of the study. It is generally prudent to ensure costs are more than adequately covered and to include administrative costs in the financial agreement. In general, local ethics committees require detailed information as to how the study will be financed.

However, new costs occasionally arise and these may need to be renegotiated with the sponsors to enable the trial to continue. Funding for drugs in development generally comes from the sponsor, however, for Phase IV studies this may be provided indirectly from the sponsor into a Trust such as in an 'educational' grant or directly from a foundation or governmental organization with an interest in a particular disease.

Details of the financial agreement should include the potential payment of volunteers, something which generally occurs only in pharmacokinetic/pharmacodynamic studies where patients are required to spend long periods of time away from home. Ethics committees will need to be clear that patient payments will not be used as an inducement to enter the study. Patients may also be refunded for expenses incurred as a result of their participation in the study, such as additional travel. Financial agreement will include:

- payment for doctors, nurses and other paramedical personnel's time

- payment for laboratory and other investigational tests and the technical assistance involved in processing these tests

- purchase of apparatus involved in the study

- the so-called 'investigator fees' paid to the university or clinic foundation

Recent FDA guidelines require investigators involved in licensing studies to provide detailed information regarding the financial relationship between themselves and the study sponsor to make it clear that they are not benefiting in a significant financial way by providing particular results.

The key to drawing up a financial agreement is to ensure that you do not sell yourself too short. Making a profit from clinical research in many national health services is important in terms of providing 'soft money' to buy additional equipment or employ additional staff within the clinic. Therefore, profit from clinical research frequently adds to the quality of the overall clinical care of all patients attending a research-based unit.

Funding Problems

Dr Pikul Moolasart, Senior Pediatrician, Head of the WHO Collaborating Center on HIV/AIDS, Bamrasnaradura Hospital, Nonthaburi, Thailand

We have a pool of trained staff with a thorough working knowledge of, and adherence to, the requirements of good clinical practice. Unfortunately, for us the major problem we face is securing appropriate funding for clinical research.

The budget for our recent clinical trial was insufficient to support a large sample size, and this had knock-on effects downstream. Some subjects were unable to attend for follow-up, as the protocol dictated, because they could not afford to take the time out from work and we were not in a position to remunerate them. In this constrained setting, securing the cooperation of pharmaceutical companies is vital. We need their support to ensure the continued availability of new medicines for our patients.

Conclusions

Working as an investigator with a research sponsor involves many responsibilities. However, it can be a rewarding experience providing patients with cutting edge therapies, participating in paradigm shifting research and feeling part of the system which enables confident and informed use of approved drugs. Although the process is not a glamorous one, presenting new research data at a meeting of your specialty and immortalizing yourself in print (and on Medline) is invariably a satisfying and rewarding experience.

■ ABBREVIATIONS

ADR	adverse drug reaction
AE	adverse event
ANOVA	analysis of variance
CRF	case report form
CTM	clinical trials monitor
EBM	evidence-based medicine
EMEA	European Medical Evaluation Agency
FDA	Food and Drug Administration
GCP	good clinical practice
NIH	National Institutes of Health
IB	investigator's brochure
ICH	International Conference on Harmonization
NTN	national training number
PI	principal investigator
REC	research ethics committee
RPU	repeating publishable unit
SOP	standard operating procedure

■ INDEX

drug handling 111
funding 7, 10, 16–17, 121–123
indemnity 106–107
industry research 19–20
setting up, curricula vitae and signatures 107–111
comparative group design *see* crossover design
compliance, clinical trials 39–40
conclusions, statistical results 75–78
confidence intervals
defined 60
estimation procedures 66–67
confounding factors 52–54
see also variables
controlled trials, single- and double-blind studies,
defined 36–38
controls, clinical trial design 37
cooking, research misconduct 95–96
coordinating center, functions 23
Coordinator, responsibilities 28, 39
correlational data *see* observational data
crossover studies, clinical trial design 37–39
curriculum vitae, commercial sponsors 109

D
data collection 34–35, 50, 119
documentation 27–29
randomized controlled trials 70–71
statistical analysis 69–72
see also case report form
Declaration of Helsinki 79–81
trial subject protection and consent 105–106
documentation
data collection 27–29
essential and source documents 34
source data verification 115–116
double-blind studies, defined 37–38
drug development 104